Contents

HEALTH INDICATORS

An International Study for
the European Science Foundation

Edited by

A J Culyer

Martin Robertson · Oxford

First published in 1983
by Martin Robertson & Company Ltd.,
108 Cowley Road, Oxford OX4 1JF.

British Library Cataloguing in Publication Data

Health indicators.
1. Health
I. Culyer, A. J.
613   RA776

ISBN 0-85520 635 7

Typeset by
Cambrian Typesetters, Aldershot.
Printed and bound in Great Britain by
Billing and Sons Ltd., Worcester

Workshop Members

Professor E.M. Backett, Department of Community Health, Queen's Medical Centre, University of Nottingham, Clifton Boulevard, Nottingham NG7 2UH, England.

Dr R.D. Brittain, North Manchester General Hospital, Central Drive, Crumpsall, Manchester M8 6RL, England.

Dr B. Brorsson, Socialmedicinska Institutionen, Akademiska Sjukhuset, Uppsala, Sweden.

Professor G.W. Brown, Department of Sociology, Social Research Unit, Bedford College, University of London, 51 Harley Street, London W1N 1DD, England.

Professor A.J. Culyer (Chairman), Department of Economics and Related Studies, University of York, Heslington, York YO1 5DD, England.

Professor M. Davies, Brookdale Institute, P.O. Box 13087, Jerusalem, Israel.

Professor M. Fardeau, Laboratoire d'Economie Sociale, Université de Paris, 24 Rue du Docteur Roux, 92330 Sceaux, France.

Professor A.J. Fox, Department of Mathematics, The City University, Northampton Square, London EC1V 0HB, England.

Dr F. Hatton, INSERM, 44 Chemin de Ronde, 78110 Le Vesinet, France.

Professor C. Helberger, Fachbereich 18 WW10, Uhlandstrasse 4–5, D-1000 Berlin 2, Federal Republic of Germany.

Professor K.-D. Henke, Lehrstuhl D für Volkswirtschaftslehre, Universität Hannover, Wunstorferstrasse 14, D-3000 Hannover 19, Federal Republic of Germany.

Dr S. Hunt, Department of Community Health, Queen's Medical Centre, University of Nottingham, Clifton Boulevard, Nottingham NG7 2UH, England.

Mr J. Hurst, Senior Economic Advisor, Department of Health and

Social Security, Friar's House, 157–168 Blackfriars Road, London SE1 8EU, England.

Professor B. Jonsson, Institutet för Halso-Och Sjukvardsekonomi, Stora Södergatan 3, 222 23 Lund, Sweden.

Dr L. Karhausen, EEC, DG XII, 200 Rue de la Loi, B-1049 Bruxelles, Belgium.

Professor E. Levy, LEGOS, Université de Paris IX, Place du Maréchal de Lattre de Tassingy, 75116 Paris, France.

Dr M.G. Marmot, Department of Medical Statistics and Epidemiology, London School of Hygiene and Tropical Medicine, Keppel Street, London WC1E 7HT, England.

Professor A. Mizrahi, CREDOC, 142 Rue du Chevaleret, 75634 Paris, France.

Mr G. Mooney, Director Health Economics Research Unit, Department of Community Medicine, University Medical Buildings, Foresterhill, Aberdeen AB9 2ZD, Scotland.

Dr P. Mossé, LEST, Chemin du Coton Rouge, 13100 Aix en Provence, France.

Dr M. Nord-Larsen, Danish National Institute of Social Research, 28 Borgengade, DK–1300, Copenhagen, Denmark.

Professor Y. Nuyens, Departement Sociologie, Katholieke Universiteit Leuven, E. Van Evenstraat 2c, 3000 Leuven, Belgium.

Dr D.L. Patrick, Department of Social and Administrative Medicine, Medical School Wing D, Box 3, 208 University of North Carolina, Chapel Hill, NC 27514, USA.

Professor M. Pfaff, Internationales Institut für Empirische Sozialökonomie, Haldenweg 23, D-8901 Augsburg-Leitershofen, Federal Republic of Germany.

Professor H. Philipsen, Faculteit der Geneeskunde, Rijksuniversiteit Limburg, Postbus 616, Maastricht, Netherlands.

Dr J.-P. Pouiller, Social Indicators Unit, OECD, 2 Rue Andre Pascal, 75775 Paris, France.

Dr R. Rosser, Department of Psychiatry, Charing Cross Hospital Medical School, University of London, Fulham Palace Road, London W6 8RF, England.

Dr E. Schroeder, Institut Infratest Gesundheitsforschung, Landsbergerstrasse 338, D-8000 München 21, Federal Republic of Germany.

Professor A. Uhde, Institutt for Okonomi, Universitet Bergen, N-5014 Bergen-U, Norway.

Dr H. Verwayen, Commissie voor de Ontwikkeling van Beleidsanalyse, Postbus 20201, 2500-EE 's-Gravenhage, Netherlands.

Mr R. Weeden, Economic Advisor's Office, Department of Health and Social Security, Friar's House, 157–168 Blackfriars Road, London SE1 8EU, England.

Dr J.W. Weehuizen, Commissie voor de Ontwikkeling van Beleidsanalyse, Postbus 20201, 2500-EE 's-Gravenhage, Netherlands.

Dr R.G.A. Williams, MRC Medical Sociology Unit, University of Aberdeen, Westburn Road, Aberdeen AB9 1FX, Scotland.

Mr K.G. Wright, Institute of Social and Economic Research, University of York, Heslington, York YO1 5DD, England.

Professor J. Zerche, Forschungsinstitut für Sozialpolitik, Universität zu Köln, Albertus-Magnus-Platz, 500 Köln 41, Federal Republic of Germany.

Preface

This book is the product of a series of three workshops held at the University of York in 1979–81. The workshops (chaired by the editor) were established by the British Social Science Research Council at the initiative of the European Science Foundation with the aims of providing a synthetic account of European research to date in the field of health indicators, to assess current research needs and to make suggestions both about future directions of research in Europe and about its organisation.

The members of the workshop were all European scholars noted for their work in this territory. The introductory chapter and the set of conclusions at the end do not necessarily represent a 'consensus' view to every part of which every member of the group would wish whole-heartedly to subscribe. They are essentially the chairman's attempt to synthesize and summarize a complex field in which many disciplines, nationalities, and interests (both academic and policy-making) are represented. They are (one hopes) both more concise and structured than the customary reports of discussion at inter-national meetings.

It is hoped, therefore, to have provided a source book that will not only introduce those who are unfamiliar with it to the field but also indicate the directions taken, problems tackled, and solutions to practical problems offered, by current research in health indicators. The comprehensive bibliography will be useful to those concerned with research in health indicators whether as 'customers' or as 'suppliers' of research. The contributed chapters constitute detailed reviews of various aspects of current research. The conclusions in the final chapter are so framed as to lead to recommendations about both research directions and research organisation.

A part of the workshop's activity was devoted to the preparation of detailed accounts of the available published information on health indicators in each of the participating European countries. This material is available from the editor upon application. A small fee will be charged to cover its duplication and postage.

The editor owes a profound debt of gratitude not only to the SSRC and ESF for making the whole thing possible but also to the members of the workshop whose scholarly and courteous discussions were evidence (should any be otherwise thought lacking) that multi-disciplinary and multinational discussion *can* work and can work *well*.

Finally, and on behalf of all the workshop members, my grateful thanks to Gail Gibson, who acted as secretary and administrator for the workshop, and kept us all on our schedules, and to Barbara Dodds who typed the proceedings and who rendered my attempts to render everyone else's attempts into English into English!

A J Culyer

1

Introduction

A J CULYER

This book is primarily about research: research in the field that has become known as 'health indicators'. Underlying this research is a complex set of motivating factors. Some of these are academic; others are administrative and policy-derived. The divisions are not, of course, watertight nor are they wholly independent of one another. The resultant literature is, however, bewildering in its variety. Some is concerned with, for example, the ideas examined in the word 'health' that 'indicators' can (or ought to) 'indicate' or 'measure' or with the monitoring of patients' conditions in response to experimental development of medicines and other therapies. Some is concerned with measures to aid prognosis and epidemiological questions concerning the impact of the environment (in the widest sense) upon the health of individuals, groups and whole societies. Other literature deals with the identification of least cost methods of health service delivery or is concerned with the development of measures of need to aid budget allocations to specialties, client groups, or geographical areas. The list of examples is not exhaustive and could easily be extended. What is clear from even this limited set of examples, however, is that the focus of interest is not unique: a 'health indicator' may mean different things to different people. Consequently, the strands of research into health indicators reflect this multiplicity of interest.

Related to this is the multiplicity of academic discipline represented in the research programme. It is by no means the monopoly of the medical subjects (even including epidemiology and community medicine among them). Major contributions have come from economists, operational researchers, psychologists, sociologists and statisticians. Since not all speak the same language nor publish in the same journals, the problem of communication between researchers and of cross disciplinary intellectual fertilization arises. Major methodological questions of research design arise: single disciplinary, multidisciplinary or interdisciplinary?

The first objective is therefore to try to describe the field so as to identify perspectives, questions, and puzzles that are shared in this diversity of interest and discipline. What follows, it is hoped, will be a useful introduction to those seeking a synoptic account of what is going on. This account is supplemented by a series of papers addressing more specific issues in some depth. For those seeking a deeper initiation into the field, a careful selection from among these papers should provide useful intellectual signposts. Further supplementation is provided by the bibliography, to which this chapter, as well as the others, makes extensive reference. The heterogeneity of the sources illustrates well the disciplinary diversity of the field that was mentioned above. The bibliography is prefaced with a short list of 'classic' contributions that, in the view of the members of the workshop, constitutes the key concept-forming articles shaping the present intellectual framework of the field.

DEVELOPMENT OF THE HEALTH INDICATORS RESEARCH FIELD

One of the starting points for the accelerating interest in health indicator development was an awareness that, especially in the developed world, the conventional data collected about mortality, life expectation, and morbidity were increasingly giving a misleading impression about health trends. There was the feeling that the general trend of these data over time was not disclosing adequately the changes that were taking place (for example, that generally rising life expectancies did not measure the changing prevalence of *disabilities* in life; were not adjusted for the possibility that 'thresholds' of acceptable illness or dysfunction were falling so that the severity with which a particular statistic was viewed might be increasing at the same time as the statistic was falling; and were insufficiently sensitive as surrogates for 'health' or 'ill-health' at both the individual and more aggregated levels). These concerns are all to be found, for example, in the care of the elderly, where increasing survival on the one hand and changing family patterns, increased labour mobility, and several other changing social phenomena on the other, raised questions about both the welfare of the elderly and how society should respond in its provision of alternative modes of care and support for this client group. There nevertheless remains an unquestionable role for the use of population-based mortality statistics in, for example, epidemiological studies (chapter 9).

Another starting point lay outside the topic of health itself: there has been a general increase of interest in developing a system of social accounts that would transcend the traditional (though in fact only twentieth century) economic measures of regional and national well-being by incorporating indices or indicators of other aspects of life. This 'social indicators' movement has grown apace and is manifest in the recent publications of several governments and in the ambitious programme of indicator development mounted by OECD. Clearly, health indicators are a part of this. So, in addition to the research impetus coming from those working in the health field who felt increasingly unhappy with the data available to them, another impetus came from outside the health field. There has been a rapid convergence of these two groups.

A third starting point lay in the more disaggregated aspects of epidemiology and the clinical practice of medicine. The development of a sophisticated method of trials for the measurement of the efficacy and effectiveness of procedures has generated, as a part of that same process, a need for, and a set of methodologies for handling outcome measurement. Such an interest in health indicators (or indices as they are more usually termed in this genre, though the distinction is one without any real difference) characteristically focuses on disaggregated populations, that is specific client groups (for example, the elderly), groups at risk (for example, workers in industry), or groups undergoing specific procedures (for example, patients suffering head injuries). A special type of aggregation problem has, however, received particular attention here: the problem of aggregating scaled *components* of 'health' into a single (usually numerical) indicator. These developments are the most sophisticated aspect of current research and are reviewed in detail in later chapters. The general development here has evinced a trend away from the traditional bio-medical measures of signs and symptoms in clincial practice (though these remain obviously important for some purposes) towards the *consequences* of disease in terms of ability to live and plan one's life satisfactorily. This approach leads naturally and directly to a consideration of the ultimate objectives of social policy in matters relating to health.

These three points of departure characterise the bulk of the present research effort. They clearly interract: scaling and the problems of developing composite indicators are an aspect of aggregate indicator developments as well as the disaggregated. They are also multidisciplinary: for example much of the pioneering work in scaling was developed by sociologists (for example, Guttman 1944), and in devising methods of combining components by operational researchers (for example, Torrance 1970) or economists (for example, Wolfson 1974, Culyer, Lavers, Williams 1971) or joint work by multidisciplinary terms (for example, Rosser and Watts 1971, Bush, Chen and Patrick 1972).

It may fairly be said that the territory now constitutes a *research programme* in which a variety of experimental techniques have been developed from several disciplines, issues of fact, analysis and value can be separated and analysed and which has begun to result in changes and new developments in the routine collection of statistical data as well as the type of data gathered for specific one-off purposes.

The rest of this introductory chapter is divided into the following heads:

'Health' and 'indicators'. This section will explore the various meanings attached to each noun: the state or condition of health (or ill-health) and its associations with disease, social and cultural factors, and so on; and the measures (which need not be in the form of numerical statistics) that purport to provide empirical counterparts to the various conceptions of health.

Disciplines. This section will look at the perspectives of the various disciplines involved in health indicators research and discuss their complementarities and the desirability of multi and interdisciplinary research.

Cause and effect. This section will investigate some of the problems that arise in associating independent variables like health services, environmental, economic and social factors with the dependent variable 'health'.

Customers. This section will identify the needs of a variety of possible customers for the output of health indicators research and discuss the implications for the kind of research undertaken.

Aggregation, values and ethics. This section will introduce the complex difficulties that arise in two types of aggregation: aggregating items of information about an individual into a single indicator and aggregating health information about individuals across groups of individuals. Aggregation can both create and destroy information: an appropriate balance has to be found. Aggregation also raises ethical issues concerning the weights to be applied to the entities being aggregated and the legitimate uses to which aggregate information may be put. Other value issues include questions concerning the values underlying the very concept of 'health' itself, questions about what to include and exclude from a health indicator, and questions to do with assigning money values to health outcomes such as may be used (or at least implied) in the judgements that have to be made about whether particular programmes of prevention, cure, or care are 'worth' their cost.

'Health' and 'Indicators'

The idea of a health indicator is deceptively simple. The simple aspect of it is that a description such as 'able to work' or 'better than yesterday', or a statistic such as a mortality rate, incidence of disease, or score on a psychometric scale, *indicates* a state of health. More usually it is intended to indicate *changes* in a state of health (whether of an individual or group) and therefore requires some quantitative element. Minimally it is usually required to convey information about more or less 'health' in comparisons across individuals or groups (cross-sections) or of the same or similar individuals or groups through time (longitudinal or time-series).

The simplicity, however, rapidly evaporates as one confronts the obvious questions: what is this state called 'health' (or 'ill-health') and is the proposed indicator a *good* indicator of 'health'/'ill-health'? In each case the answer appears to depend on the context in which the question is being asked (see chapter 2).

One common approach has been to see health as the absence of disease where 'disease' connotes a medical concept of abnormality in pathological function with an associated set of symptoms, prognoses and (in some cases) remedial measures. It is closely associated with diagnosis: assigning a medical label to the condition. This so-called 'medical model' evidently has important uses, particularly in the scientific practice of modern medicine.

It also, however, has its limitations. If, for example, one is concerned with the question of why individuals consult a doctor, then it appears that an experiential concept of health or ill-health is more appropriate: *feeling* 'ill' (experiencing pain, discomfort, restriction on activity and similar subjective or objective phenomena) may be more important. It is possible for someone to 'feel ill' without having a disease. It is similarly possible for someone to have a disease without 'feeling ill' (the condition may be presymptomatic or asymptomatic).

The 'medical model' has also proved difficult to adapt for the purposes of including psychiatric and emotional disorders.

The medical model has been particularly objected to by those having an emotional commitment to preventive rather than restorative medicine and by those who emphasise the natural propensity of the human body to 'heal' itself without interventions that are sometimes extremely invasive and that themselves may do damage to the health ('medical model' variety) of the individual.

The 'medical model' is also unsatisfactory from a 'social' perspective. For example, suppose one were concerned to reduce the prevalence of 'feeling ill' in the community. There is abundant evidence (see Field 1976) that the predisposing factors include a subtle set of socially determined elements. An extreme example of clinical disease that was not regarded as 'being ill' in the relevant community is pinto (dichromic spirochetosis), a skin disease that is so prevalent among some South American tribes that the few single men *not* suffering from it were regarded as pathological to the point of being excluded from marriage (Ackerknecht 1947).

Zola (1966) noted an inverse correlation between the perceived significance of a disability or symptom and its prevalence and a positive correlation between disability or symptom and dominant cultural values. Low back pain is a common phenomenon among women in low social classes in the West: it is not considered symptomatic of any disease but part of their everyday existence. 'Tiredness' is not only a ubiquitous physical sign but a correlate of a vast set of physical diseases. Yet in a study of students who kept a diary noting all bodily states and conditions, tiredness, though often noted, was rarely cited as a cause for concern. Attending school, and having a peer group that stressed hard work and achievement, caused tiredness almost to become an end in itself: proof positive they were conforming to the accepted norm rather than an indication of 'something wrong'. By contrast, where work is arduous and not in itself gratifying, tiredness becomes a matter for concern and perhaps medical consultation. Nausea is a common and treatable phenomenon of pregnancy yet Margaret Mead (1950) found no evidence of morning sickness among the Arapesh and suggested this was due to their almost complete denial that a child exists until shortly before birth. In another setting, where existence of life is dated from conception, nausea is the external sign, hope and proof of pregnancy.

Expectations, social customs, financial incentives, and a variety of other factors seem to be major determinants of behaviour. They also affect the social significance attached to both 'disease' and 'illness'. They also affect the relationships of individuals with one another and the medical professions: the 'legitimating' role of the physician in certifying someone as 'sick' and prescribing 'treatments' affects the legitimate claims they may make upon their family, work colleagues, and so on and defines a set of expected responses on the part of the 'sick' person (doing what the doctor says, trying to 'get better' and so on). This special 'sick role' has been analysed particularly subtly by Parsons (1951).

Besides the pathological concept of health as absence of 'disease', and the sociological concept of health as the absence of 'illness', there is the idealised conception of 'positive' health advocated by the World Health Organisation as 'a state of complete physical, mental and social well-being'. While some have felt drawn to this idea it has for the most part met with a cool reception. It is arguably far too broad an idea, corresponding more to social philosophers' conceptions of 'welfare' than to 'health'. Moreover, whether such a state can actually be described in a non-relativist fashion (let alone measured) seems to be in doubt: if 'health' is conceived as a continuum of states of which one extreme is 'perfect health', it seems both analytically more manageable and practically more relevant to focus on the in-between states and on improvements (movements towards the state of 'perfect health') than upon the extreme state itself which may be unattainable and even unimaginable.

Cutting across these various abstractions is a more pragmatic tradition defining health (or ill-health) in terms of an eclectic set of 'characteristics' of individuals. These might include functional capacity (ability to perform physical activities), pain, emotional state or, indeed, anything else deemed relevant for the purposes in mind. This has been the characteristic view taken by researchers in health indicators.

The 'characteristics' approach does not at all exclude the insights and leverage on real problems to be gained from the alternatives discussed above. Insights derived by applying the 'medical model', for example, lead one to seek associations between the signs and symptoms that are important guides for medical intervention and the characteristics that may have greater significance for the quality of life. If, for example, one were to judge the former as being primarily of importance in the clinical management of a case, the latter may be judged of greater importance in determining the priority in terms of resource availability to be given to cases of that type. Insights from the 'characteristics' approach may likewise feed back into medical management of disease. A good example occurs in a field that is neither 'care' nor 'cure' but has come to be termed 'rescue': life or death situations where a doctor, usually having highly specialized equipment and skills, has to determine whether or not to intervene in the case of a patient who can be expected to die in the near future without intervention. Intensive care, oncology, renal dialysis and transplantation, intracranial surgery all entail procedures that are of the 'rescue' variety. Whom should one treat supposing one cannot treat all eligible cases? Should one treat when the prognosis is very poor indeed even with treatment? Part of the answer must lie in the expected outcome of treating a patient having the presenting condition. In many rescue cases the outcome cannot be expected to restore the individual to anything like the state of health prior to the disease. Many neurosurgeons would maintain that survival after severe brain damage may be judged a disaster both by victim and his or her family. If so this requires the measurement of the later social aspects of recovery and their linking with early symptomatic evidence to enable good prognoses to determine what action (if any) should be taken when the patient presents in a state of trauma.

The 'characteristics' approach relates to the sociological view of illness by virtue of the fact that the selection of 'characteristics' as relevant or not will be determined by their importance in the social, economic, and cultural circumstances of the society in question. Apple (1960) among others found that whether or not an experience is interpreted by a lay person as symptomatic of disease depends on its novelty, the extent to which it interferes with ordinary activities and the person's independence of others. Since novelty depends upon local incidence and prevalence, and both 'ordinary' activities and the interdependencies between people vary much from society to society, it is clear that the social element in the selection of characteristics is all-pervading. This contingent element in the 'characteristics' approach applies not only at the broad social level but carries on down to the particular circumstances of the individual: life-styles, job and family circumstances, and so on. In a real sense a one-legged professor is less handicapped than a one-legged footballer; a deaf machine-tool operator than a deaf composer; a blind musician than a blind painter.

While it may be hazardous to identify any firm trend in a field of study as young as health indicators, the treatment of health as a set of characteristics does seem to be emerging as a dominant approach. This raises further important questions concerning the *selection* of relevant characteristics. In empirical studies that use health indicators as a part of a behavioural account enabling, say, *explanation* of past patterns of behaviour, or prediction of future patterns, the ultimate determining factor will be empirical: the relevant characteristics are those that as a matter of fact seem to account for the behaviour in question. In normative studies, where the health indicator is going to be used for purposes that logically entail an ethical value or set of values (for example, 'resources ought to go to those areas where ill-health is worst') then quite different criteria for selection will be used. These issues are discussed extensively in chapter 3 and will crop up several times again in this chapter.

The 'content validity' of health indicators has been much discussed (for example, by Kaplan *et al.* 1976). Essentially 'content validity' is concerned with the question whether the health indicator *really* measures what it purports to measure, that is, 'health'. With approaches that define an abstract concept of health and consider the indicator as a more or less adequate empirical surrogate or proxy for that conceptual variable, the question of content validity is evidently real. With the characteristics approach, however, the problem evaporates. The indicator incorporating various characteristics *is* 'health' (or 'ill-health'). One may ask (in a behavioural context) if the indicator is a good predictor (say, of the utilization of health services). One may ask (in a normative context) if the indicator embodies acceptable values, if the indicator is sufficiently sensitive to changes in the parameters that may affect it or if the indicator contains logical inconsistencies within itself (such as combination A of characteristics being recorded as worse than combination B, and combination B being worse than A). But the question whether the indicator is a good measure of *health* is meaningless. The appropriate question is whether the right characteristics are included (requiring a set of value judgements in the normative case and a set of empirical judgements in the predictive case).

The foregoing will suggest a great variety in the descriptions and numerical measures that may be considered to be health indicators. For some purposes familiar, if crude, data relating to mortality may be useful, perhaps classified according to cause of death as in the 'medical model'. At the opposite extreme measures exist that scale the ability of elderly individuals in residential homes to perform basic physical functions of everyday living. The range is immense and each type of measure will normally have its uses. The unity of health indicators research is characterized by great diversity!

Disciplines

Both the medical and the social sciences are beset by disciplinary *amours propres*, interdisciplinary rivalry, and crossdisciplinary incomprehension. Health indicators research is characterized by the presence within it of several disciplines. Their productive mutual existence needs supporting.

It is useful to keep in mind a distinction made by Williams (1979) between an 'area of study' and a 'mode of thinking'. The former connotes a set of topics — empirical, social, conceptual, and the like to be comprehended and resolved. The latter denotes the disciplinary conventions, theories, and so on that may be brought to bear on the topics. If as a shorthand we use 'topic' and 'discipline' to refer to these two sets of considerations we have a useful way of exploring some of the complex interrelationships that can arise.

While many topics are traditionally associated with particular disciplines (for example, the discipline 'economics' is traditionally associated with the descriptive topic 'the economy') there is no logically compelling reason for regarding such associations as immutable or exclusive: the economic topic of inflation is, for example, not merely the preserve of the *discipline* of economics: political science, psychology and sociology also have illuminating things to say about it. Nor is health a topic exclusively for medicine: other disciplines also have much to contribute.

To give more substance to these claims, consider figure 1.1. This contains a list of disciplines (in alphabetical order) and a list of topics relating to treatment of duodenal ulcer disease. The items in each list are rather arbitrary but serve to illustrate the point. The lines connecting the disciplines and topics indicate that the discipline in question (the discipline, not the profession) has an intellectual apparatus capable of application to the topics to which it is connected or, in entirely symmetrical fashion, topics some aspect of which requires an input from the discipline indicated.

The general topic of 'health' likewise 'belongs to' all of the listed disciplines (and others too no doubt). Since it is often the case that disciplines are associated traditionally with particular topics figure 1.1 dramatically reveals that traditional associations are no more than that — they are conventional, not logical, in nature. Accordingly, it is wrong to suppose that only, say, medicine is concerned with health and ill-health or economics with finance. Nearly all of the topics that may lie inside 'health' are multidisciplinary research topics. This does not necessarily imply that all, or even most, research in the field of 'health' should be jointly prosecuted by a multidisciplinary team. But there will be many problems that will be usefully tackled by a joint team and, depending on the nature of the work being done, it will always be sensible to maintain an awareness

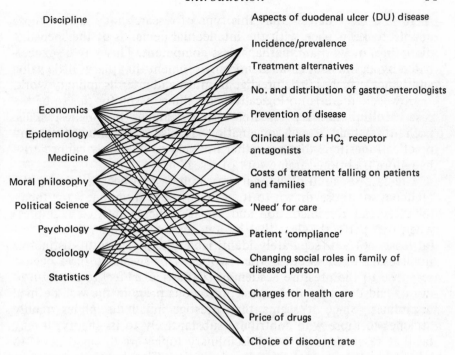

FIG 1.1 *Relationship between disciplines and treatments*

of what it is that other disciplines have contributed, or could contribute. Moreover, in the training of researchers in these topics it may sometimes be useful for more than one set of disciplinary skills to be acquired.

With such multidisciplinary topics it is important to seek to avoid 'border disputes' between disciplines fearing the 'invasion' of 'their' territory by others. This is best done by acquiring an informed awareness of the mode of thinking each has to offer and how they may mutually complement one another.

Multidisciplinary research is often contrasted with interdisciplinary research. If the former usually connotes 'teams' of individuals having, as individuals, the particular skills associated with a discipline, the latter usually connotes one individual with multiple skills, or a team of such multiple-skilled individuals. Both types are often regarded (by traditional specialists) with suspicion: the single discipline person in a multidisciplinary team because of the reduced level of specialist peer criticism he or she may have; the multidisciplinary individual because of the 'jack of all trades — master of none' tag. In each case there is a clear danger that this type of research may attract those unable to keep pace with the intellectual demands of the specialist disciplines or who are, perhaps, less competent. This may be exacerbated by an intellectual/academic environment that places little value and hence attaches little prestige to multi and interdisciplinary work.

However, there is no logically compelling reason for this to be the case. Multidisciplinary research often demands the highest skills, both of technique and imagination. It also raises intellectual and practical questions that are either unlikely to or simply cannot arise in a more traditional framework of research.

The case for multidisciplinary research has not been helped by the tendency of those drawn to it to invent new 'disciplines' for themselves (social administration and social medicine are two examples) when it is perfectly clear that by any reasonable canon they are not (at least, not yet) separately identifiable disciplines, with distinctive intellectual or theoretical frameworks. This seems to have been a response to the pressure academics (in particular) feel to conform to norms laid down by their most prestigious peers in the well-defined disciplines. Since it seems that prestige in all disciplines mainly attaches to those who contribute substantively to its theory, it may be that researchers in multidisciplinary topics are doomed never to rise higher than top of the second division. This, however, would be to deny that intense exposure to other disciplines cannot yield insights that may in turn feed back into the process of intellectual discovery in the mainstream of the discipline. Only a few may be able to do this. But only a few make such contributions anyway.

What is needed is the creation and nurturing of a sympathetic intellectual environment in which researchers in explicitly multidisciplinary topics can work without severing contact with their traditional mainstream peers and where the commitment is to the highest standards of research. In the end, prestige and honour will go to those with good ideas and/or capable of *applying* good ideas imaginatively and effectively.

A common restraint that has been placed upon multidisciplinary researchers is that the outlets for publication of their work are, by and large, controlled by representatives of single disciplines. Health indicators research illustrates this well: a high proportion of the references in the bibliography in this volume are not in multidisciplinary journals. This imposes a useful discipline, and protects work in the topic from the incompetent and second rate. A disadvantage, however, is that the topic (health indicators) may be regarded by editors as of rather minor interest to the bulk of their readership.

Hence, while it seems there is no pressing need for a specialist journal for the topic 'health indicators' the existence of topic-related journals, dealing with the broader set of issues in health services research, is necessary. Where appropriate, however, researchers in this multi-disciplinary field should also publish in the discipline-related journals and other outlets directed at disciplinary specialists. The burden of proof of their 'respectability' lies with them. They should not shirk its implications.

Inherent in this multidisciplinary characterization of health indicators is the risk that research will become fragmented and contacts hard to establish across disciplinary frontiers, partly because researchers from one discipline may not understand what researchers from others have to offer, partly because there may be hostility (a hostility that typically evaporates once understanding is acquired) and partly because, even if the former two problems could be resolved, one simply may not know the individuals, centres of work, networks, and so on that would make crossdisciplinary information flows and even joint research a practical possibility. Again, the case for creating such means of communication and information diffusion is clear and the burden of making it lies with the researchers in the field. The research councils and other research sponsoring foundations have an obligation to respond positively to well-designed proposals for increasing communication between researchers.

Cause and Effect

It is useful to see the place of health indicators in the wider context of health services research by considering figure 1.2. This depicts a familiar set of issues relating to health as an inter-related group. In essence, the 'processes' (indicated significantly by the black box) that affect health for good or ill are seen as embracing resource inputs; patients, individuals or communities; and environmental factors. Process itself refers not only to processes internalized in familiar health care institutions like hospitals and general practices but all processes by which an individual's health is affected – often in ways that are either not understood very well or not understood at all. The environment is taken to include working conditions, familial relations and structures, costs of access to services, health information, social conventions, and a host of social, attitudinal and technological features that may affect health.

For many, the idea of 'health' is to be interpreted essentially as an outcome of this variety of processes. The ellipse labelled 'outcomes' is in such cases concerned with questions relating to the conceptualization and measurement of health, or changes in health, as a response to changes in environmental factors, inputs, individual demands and perceptions, and organizational forms. On this view an important aspect of the development of indicators is naturally the invention of measures of health that can be related to the determining and predisposing variables in other ellipses via an understanding of the complex of processes. In this way information is generated that might inform policy makers, administrators, doctors, and the like, or elucidate an understanding of what determines what and how changes in one aspect may change another (see especially chapter 8).

The idea of health as an outcome, though underlying all approaches to the conceptualization and measurement of health, is not, however, immutable. For some purposes what will be needed might be indicators of prevalence and/or incidence of specified diseases. For others, some indicator of psychological and social functioning might be desired. For others indicators of subjective perceptions would be appropriate. Yet others focus on the distinctions and interplay between impairment, disability and handicap. In each case what is shared in common is that the indicator is taken as a measure corresponding more or less faithfully to an underlying concept of health, ill-health, 'deprivation' or need. The nature of that underlying concept ought to be determined by the nature of the question being

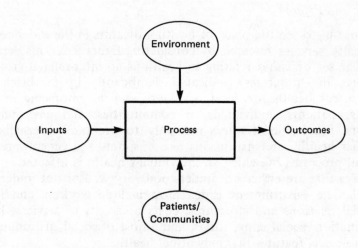

FIG 1.2 *Health issues as inter-related group*

asked or the problem being tackled. For some questions the indicator will need to be felt to be a reasonably complete measure of the attributes deemed relevant. For others it may be regarded merely as a useful 'tracer' or 'surrogate' whose value (content validity) would lie in the extent to which it was believed to correlate with other underlying features that were the true objects of ultimate interest. Other foci of interest lie in various objectives like prevention or cure of ill-health, or in making compensations for its consequences.

Few studies are so all-embracing as to investigate the interraction of all components of figure 1.2. Indeed, so little is known about the content of the 'black box' in many cases that this is frequently not possible. This is certainly the case with highly aggregated information of the sort shown in table 1.1. Here the first four columns represent species of inputs that are 'transformed' by some process (not specified) into the 'outputs' of the last three columns through the mediation of varying historical, environmental, demographic (and so on) factors specific to each country. Such exercises may be more useful for the questions they pose rather than those they answer. But even this modest claim should not be underestimated. It was, for example, the widespread view that 'output' data of the sort represented in table 1.1 were grossly inadequate representations of output (and also probably more sensitive to historical and environmental factors than health service inputs) that provided, as we have seen, one major motivation for the development of more refined health indicators.

Whether the case is one of broad international comparisons at one extreme or evaluation of specific medical procedures, preventive programmes, alternative modes of care, environmental control and so on at the other, the problem of placing content in the 'black box' cannot be resolved until acceptable measures of outcome are produced. This is the problem of identifying efficacy and effectiveness in epidemiology (where efficacy relates to the effects of a procedure on outcome under carefully controlled, ideal, conditions and effectiveness refers to the effects under normal operational conditions). It is the object of behavioural model building in economics, sociology and political science. It is also an area of ignorance that has to be removed if economic analysis of efficiency (cost-benefit and cost-effectiveness analysis) is to be applied to health services. This is the single most important area of research in the health services field, for if it is true as many have asserted (White 1982 is typical) that only about 15 per cent of medical procedures are known to be effective in terms of their impact on health or welfare, then we lack even the basic know-

TABLE 1.1 *Health Service Resources and Results: International Comparisons 1974 or Near Date*[1]

Country	Per capita total expenditure on health US$[2]	% Trend GDP[3]	Doctors (per 10,000 1974)	Nurses (per 10,000 1974)	Life expectancy at age 1 M	F	Perinatal mortality (per 1,000 live births)	Maternal mortality (per 100,000 births)
Australia	308	6.5	13.9	54.1	68.5	75.4	22.4	11.3
Canada	408	6.8	16.6	57.8	69.7	77.0	17.7	10.8
Finland	265	5.8	13.3	46.0	66.8	75.7	17.1	10.6
France	352	6.9	13.9	23.7	69.5	77.1	18.8	24.0
Italy	191	6.0	19.9	7.8	70.0	76.0	29.6	42.4
Japan	166	4.0	11.6	16.1	70.8	76.0	18.0	38.3
Netherlands	312	7.3	14.9	22.5	71.2	76.9	16.4	10.3
Norway	270	5.6	16.5	46.4	71.4	77.7	16.8	3.3
Sweden	416	7.3	16.2	58.6	72.0	77.4	14.1	2.7
USA	491	7.4	16.5	40.4	68.0	75.6	24.8	15.2
W. Germany	336	6.7	19.4	27.6	68.6	74.9	23.2	45.9
England and Wales			13.1	33.7	69.5	75.6	21.3	13.0
Scotland	212	5.2	16.1	45.6	67.7	74.0	22.7	21.5
N. Ireland			15.3	36.6	67.0	73.6	25.9	17.1

Sources: Organisation for Economic Co-operation and Development *Public Expenditure on Health*, Paris, 1977, Table 1.

McKinsey & Co., *International Comparisons of Health Needs and Health Services*, 1978.

Irving B. Kravis, Alan W. Heston and Robert Summers, "Real GDP per capita for more than one hundred countries", *Economic Journal*, June 1978, Table 4.

Notes: [1] There are a number of caveats concerning the figures in this table. Details are given in the sources listed.

[2] The column is indicative rather than definitive: it has been derived by multiplying per cent of trend GDP spent on health care by actual GDP adjusted for purchasing power difference.

[3] Trend GDP is used to avoid the influence of cyclical business fluctuations on the level of output, which could distort the measured share of health expenditure in that output. For details see OECD, *Public Expenditure on Health*, Paris, 1977, page 9.

ledge for the rational, efficient and humane allocation of resources in health. We must rely instead on hunch, *ad hoc* experience, pressure from interest groups and the vagaries of ill-informed demand and supply. The application of health indicators as measures of outcome is an essential component of any attempt to understand and rearrange the contents of the 'black box'.

Just as the idea of health as an outcome is not particularly restrictive, neither is the idea of an indicator. In health studies one does not merely need indicators of health or ill-health. One may want, for example, indicators of utilization (a part of 'process'); indicators of harmful effluent emission, of attitudes, of accessibility (all parts of 'environment'); indicators of community health workers (whole time equivalents), of medical manpower (weighted by salary), and the like (all parts of 'inputs'); indicators of demographic composition, case-mix, case-complexity, and so on (all parts of 'patients/communities').

In this outline it is clear that we are locating both concepts of health and concepts of indicators within a wider conceptual framework. Some frameworks may be rather informal; others highly structured. Some simple; others complex and highly interactive. Some are designed with policy customers in mind; others are motivated solely by the search for a better understanding.

Both the idea of 'health' (or, more usually, ill-health) and that of 'indicator' are thus highly variable but the various approaches adopted by different workers in the field are determined much less by differences in any fundamental view as to what is being done than by the specific nature of the task they have set themselves. Whether the basic framework is one postulating that behaviour (utilization, adoption of sick roles, and so on) is at least in part determined by beliefs or expectations about a changing health status, or one postulating that systems, or parts of systems, should be so designed as to have the greatest impact of health, given the resources available, the idea of outcome or output is central. It is the measurement of output to which all health indicators research ultimately aspires.

Customers

The variety within the health indicators research field that has been illustrated so far is further compounded by the diversity of purposes for which indicators of health may be seen as instrumental and, hence, by the diversity of potential 'customers' for research in the topic. The issues arising are discussed in detail by Weehuizen and Klaasen, Nord-Larsen, and Uhde in chapters 5–7. They are illustrated in a policy-making context in chapter 8 and 9. Chapter 4 well illustrates the dangers of having researchers and users embodied in the same person.

A short list of the main uses of health indicators would include:

evaluation (efficacy, effectiveness and efficiency) of alternative procedures, processes, financial systems, and so on; monitoring of the same (implying the need for periodic data collection); prognosis and forecasting at the individual, group or societal level (implying the need for integration of health indicators in bio-medical, epidemiological, demographic, and other such models); investigating the environmental, occupational and life-style patterns that are associated with disease; development of other aetiological aspects of disease in the community with associated analyses of the value of presymptomatic screening and early detection; allocation of resources to and within health services and the health-affecting environment (implying integration of health indicators in economic models, systems analysis, and so on); compensation for injury, ill-health, death, and the like; incentive systems for health service personnel, patients and individuals in the community; budgeting in the health services and other sectors that affect health. In all cases, and underlining the multidisciplinary nature of the topic, health indicators need if they are to be useful to be put into a theoretical model or construct that derives from a body of thought lying outside the indicator field: for example ethics, medical science, sociology, economics, epidemiology.

A short list of the principal customers to whom health indicators may be useful in the discharge of their duties and the playing of their roles would include: health service providers (physicians, nurses, and so on); health service planners and managers; the community as consumers of care; the community as providers of care; the community as *potential* patients; the legislature (for example, in designing systems of ownership, control, accountability, liability, finance, safety). the judiciary (for example, in determining compensation or fault); international organisations and teachers. The research community is, of course, both a supplier of health indicators and itself a customer for them.

It is the clear perception of the ultimate purpose and use of a health indicator that enables the transformation of mere *data* into *information*, whether it be information required by decision makers in health services management or information required by researchers in testing scientific hypotheses. As has been noted above, there are ample data about health services (particularly in the developed world). But there has been a paucity of *information*.

Aggregation, Values and Ethics

Values impinge in two rather distinct ways upon the health indicators research programme. The first, rather general way, is that the socio-economic environment is itself a conditioning factor that affects not only the way in which policy concerns emerge and are dealt with but also affects researchers themselves: often affecting subconsciously the way in which research questions are put, whether or not particular questions get put at all, and always requiring a sceptical attitude on the part of the researcher as to whether he or she may not be infiltrating values into an apparently 'objective' or 'scientific' research task. The second arises whenever *action* is based upon health status information, necessarily entailing as it does, either the explicit or implicit weighting of alternative outcomes in terms of 'better' or 'worse' or, in cost-benefit analysis, the explicit or implicit weighting of benefits (in terms of health improvements or prevention of deterioration) against the costs of attaining them. While some of these value questions are extremely broad, others cry out for expression in terms of a numeraire index of value — for which role money is the most popular contender. Both sets of issues are of crucial importance. Neither is receiving much attention from researchers.

Values conditioning research. The sorts of issue arising in the first type of value question, concerning the importance of research, are extremely difficult to set out in an orderly fashion. There is the danger that researchers become excessively attracted by sophistication for its own sake, to the detriment of developing usable measures for policy purposes, without sufficient regard to the costs of using proposed indicators, and with the risk of bringing into (professional) disrepute conventional (and often useful) measures of infant, maternal, and the like mortality. These dangers require a particular kind of responsibility and self-discipline on the part of researchers in the field. Close and continuing contact with potential 'customers' is probably the best defence against such dangers and it is important that links between policy 'customers' and researchers be strengthened (and in some cases established) to protect against them. Such contact is also a useful protection against the excessive separation of theory and application in health indicators research. It also has its dangers. Mossé, in chapter 4, comments on the relative lack of sophistication of French work in indicators and the (related) excessive closeness of customers and researchers. It is also important, of course, that the demand for quick (and often 'dirty') results from policy makers should not distort the balance of research 'too much' away from thoroughgoing scholarly work. What the optimal combination of the two should be is not, however, readily identifiable. Nor should it need adding that governmental policy makers should not be the sole judges of the relevance of the applications! However, it seems clear that, given the propensity for many medical technologies to gain a rapid (and often costly) diffusion prior to the full evaluation of their effectiveness and efficiency, the need for early 'quick and dirty' studies is ever present. Such studies demand *more* rather than less skill on the part of researchers since the assumptions on which they are based and the interpretations reasonably to be put on their results require a high order of professional experience and judgement.

A second, more insidious, danger is that health indicators become unconsciously couched in terms of an underlying set of values reflecting the ethics of a dominant ideology: for example, ability to participate in the labour force (men only!), to do housework (women only!), to perform certain specific social roles sanctioned and approved by society. The assertion here is not so much that indicators should *not* reflect a dominant ideology (it is easy to argue that often it is entirely appropriate that they should) as that researchers should at least be aware of what they are doing so that their results are not rendered useless by an inability to respond, say, to *changes* in dominant ideologies or by an inapplicability to 'sub-cultures' that coexist with the dominant ideology, or to different institutional contexts (for example, ones with different degrees of governmental intervention and regulation in the health territory). These, and related issues, are discussed in chapter 11.

Values needed in research. Many researchers recognize and specifically identify the necessity for making value judgements of the second variety, particularly in designing composite health indicators. This gives rise to a series of value considerations. One is: who should be making these value judgements? A classic case arises in 'trading-off' different dimensions in a composite index (as well as in selecting dimensions in the first place). The potential list of persons who should make such judgements is long and includes researchers themselves, clients whose welfare will be affected by the use of the index, experts like doctors, health service planners and administrators, politicians. There is relatively little research tackling the issues that arise here.

There is another set of ethical issues arising from the empirical implementation of a theoretical index: this includes questions of privacy and protection of the individuals (or groups) whose health is being measured as well as the classic questions of medical ethics concerning the legitimacy of particular types of experiment (for example, in trials of clinical or preventive procedures).

There is another, extremely under-researched, area where health indicators research and political philosophy interrelate. This concerns, for example, questions of social equity that must be regarded as no less important than the effectiveness/efficiency questions characterizing the bulk of the work currently under way. For example, questions of distributive justice in health policy have commonly been associated with deriving justifications for propositions concerning 'equality of access' to health services or 'equality of opportunity to lead a healthy life'. Distributive concerns such as these may both *affect* concepts of health (and hence health indicators) and, as research results are achieved, *be affected by* the availability of reliable and valid measures.

Yet another set of value issues concerns the value to be attached to health itself: its relation with other moral objectives (for example, whether tradeable-off or lexically prior), its relation with other components of 'well-being' in a 'social welfare function' and the danger of elevating good health to a status it does not deserve and that, through lack of proper consideration, implicitly relegates other moral pursuits to a subordinated status.

The set of issues concerning the valuation of health states is not logically independent of the matters mentioned above but tends to arise for explicit attention within the research programme and has therefore received greater, if nonetheless scant, attention. Their character is more technical and less philosophical than the foregoing and they tend to arise in the context of 'how' rather than 'whether' or 'by whom' value judgements have to be or should be made.

One set of value issues here relates to matters concerning *how* (as distinct from *by whom*) relative weights are to be assigned to components of an individual's health status in the derivation of a composite index. Such issues are described later (see especially chapter 3) and the techniques used to deal with them are there discussed. Nor can they be side-stepped where mortality is deemed an adequate outcome indicator (see chapter 9) or where cumulative scaling is possible (see chapter 10) since these measures also implicitly embody weights — cardinal in the case of life and death (where the weights are 0 to 1) and ordinal in the case of cumulative indices.

Another issue, but one that has received less attention, concerns the manner in which different *individuals'* health characteristics are to be aggregated in an index of the health status of a group. This is clearly an aspect of distributional equity but it has not been explicitly faced up to in the health indicators literature, the usual procedure being rather on the face of it rather arbitrary: assigning equal weights to each individual.

Another set of issues arises in the assignment of values to health outcomes for comparison with the costs of attaining those outcomes. Oddly enough progress here, which is mainly the result of economists' work, has been made in what may be thought the hardest issue of all, the valuation of life. The usual procedure has been to use one of three methods: decision-makers' revealed preferences; the human capital approach (present value of suitably adjusted earned income streams); and the *ex ante* valuation of reduced risks of death. The judgement seems widespread that progress in the valuation (in money terms) of changes in health status will proceed best when health status itself is better measured, but it is easily argued that conceptually there is no reason for this sequential approach — at least at a sufficiently general level of conceptualization — and, in any case, there are ample measures already available at this stage in the life of the research programme for experimentation with techniques addressed to this question. These issues are also discussed throughout this book (see especially chapter 12).

Related to the valuation of health outcomes for comparison with cost is the question of whether increments of health are to be regarded as subject to the widely used principle of declining marginal value (utility). This has both moral aspects (*ought* it to be so regarded?) and behavioural aspects (do people act as though it actually were the case?). Neither issue has received much attention.

A characteristic of all the remarks made in this section has been the relative lack of research attention given to issues of value. These deficiencies indicate a respect in which the research programme has become unbalanced to date and future developments will need to redress the balance lest an increasing technical sophistication in the art of health indicator construction take place in a moral and political vacuum. This is an aspect of health indicator research to which the social scientists should be able to contribute a good deal.

2

Concepts of
Health and Illness

ERNST SCHROEDER

INTRODUCTION

Health indicators describe and measure different states of health of individuals and groups of individuals. In developing such indicators, an inductive or a deductive approach may be chosen (Jazairi 1976). The inductive approach starts from the requirements and methodological problems of the users of health indicators. The deductive approach refers to a theoretical concept of what is meant by the state of health, by health and illness. This paper deals only with concepts of health and illness. It is a rather incomplete summary of definitions found in the present literature. Reviewing these publications, the following questions, which are important for the development of health indicators, have been kept in mind: can health on the one hand and illness on the other be defined and distinguished to represent alternative classifications of states of health? Can further subclassifications be defined within 'health' and 'illness'? Can they be arranged at least on an ordinal scale to mark different states of health? Can the state of health of groups of individuals be described as the aggregate of the status of individuals?

THE PLURALITY OF THE CONCEPTS OF HEALTH AND ILLNESS-OVERVIEW

Even today a universally valid, comprehensive and accepted definition of health and illness does not exist (Schaefer 1978). Definitions found in both the early and the more recent literature reflect the state of knowledge of the relevant sciences (clinical and social medicine, psychology, sociology, jurisprudence and so on). Moreover, both the definitions and the phenomena defined are affected by the power structure of a society and particular groups have particular interests in the process of providing definitions and measures of social phenomena. Definitions of health and illness are therefore part and parcel of societies, cultures and epochs (Schaefer 1976). For example, in medicine, the classification of different diseases originated from growing knowledge about their aetiology, their pathogenesis, symptoms and therapies. This process has also depended upon the development of new laboratory technology. Most definitions, mainly coming from the industrialized world, relate to clinical-scientific medicine. This reflects the strong (almost monopolistic) professional interest that doctors have in the definition process — at both the societal as well as the individual level.

The broadening of the concept of health, mainly promoted by the WHO with its definition of health as a state of complete physical, mental, and social well-being (not merely the absence of disease or infirmity) had the very pragmatic purpose of proposing an ideal objective, that countries with very different cultures, economic backgrounds and health systems could nevertheless use to guide their health policy.

It is generally accepted that health and illness in the extreme can be clearly distinguished, but there exist areas of discretion, where individuals, organisms or parts thereof cannot be assigned unambiguously to the one side or the other. Health and illness have therefore often been defined separately, but very often one term is related to the other, so that circular definitions result.

Attempts to narrow the area of discretion between health and illness have lead some to the definition of health as a norm (Van Engelhardt 1978). Illness is the negative deviation of the status or behaviour of an individual, organism or part thereof from a norm. This norm can be a statistical measure, characteristic of an average group of people (of given age and sex) or organisms or parts thereof. It can be an ideal principle that may actually exist but does not, like a statistical norm, depend on the frequency of events: for example an individual's normal state, or whatever an individual considers is meant by 'healthy' (Ueberla 1979). Finally, there is always debate concerning what is supposed to be the norm. Therefore, at least in the area of discretion, illness is more socially than naturally determined (Von Ferber 1978).

Besides attempts to define and distinguish between health and illness, other conceptual problems are related to their genesis. Illness is always the result of an interference that has acted on an individual, organism or part thereof. In the classical medical disease model every specific disease, manifested in specific signs and symptoms, is caused by specific pathogens 'hosted' in the patient's body (Illsley 1977), and is due to specific pathological processes in the biochemical functions of the body. The emphasis on a specific aetiology leads to emphasis on specific individual disease-oriented therapies.

This engineering approach in the medical care process has been critized by Szasz (1961), among other, mainly in relation to mental illnesses. In the view of these critics mental illnesses are due to interpersonal interactions and not to intra-individual processes. Mental deviations arise in social settings, where individuals with interpersonal problems are forced into deviancy (notwithstanding the problem of defining normal behaviour).

The aetiological model has been extended not only into the psychiatric, but also into the sociomedical and psychosomatic side to include all states of health. Multicausal/multifactorial models of this kind define health and illness as the result of the interaction between:

(1)   behaviour patterns and those factors that determine them: socialization, group conventions, acceptance of social roles, and the like;
(2)   the reaction of the individual to these influences;
(3)   external attacks to the body and organism, for example, infections, accidents, stress.

All these factors are influenced by congenital conditions, for example, congenital deformations and impairments (Lueth 1979).

From the point of view of current medical sociology, health and illness are judgements about physical and socio-physical phenomena. Labelling the 'state of health' of a person 'healthy' or 'ill' is socially defined. 'Health status is a label agreed between an individual and others, with whom he interacts, his status definers' (Stacey 1977).

The judgements are made according to the normative and cognitive perspectives of several groups or individuals (Von Ferber 1978): the affected individual himself at some particular point in his life-cycle; some reference person in the individual's own environment, whether medical layman, medical practitioner or family doctor – the community of medical scientists; social policy as is reflected in social security arrangements voted by legislative authorities; the community of scientists with a preventive medical orientation. Each of these sets of people judges from different standpoints depending on their perceptions, interests and obligations.

In the following sections concepts of illness from the viewpoints of different individuals are outlined, each describing the state of health in different dimensions. For each dimension specific variables or components are indicated that might be used to describe different levels of health.

DIMENSIONS OF ILLNESS

Illness from the Layman's Viewpoint

From the viewpoint of the layman illness is characterized by the following variables:

(1) disturbances in his condition, that is physical complaints (for example, pain, fever, feebleness) and mental complaints (for example, anxiety, inability to concentrate);
(2) impairment of physical functioning;
(3) impairment of normal behaviour (restriction of usual daily activities in consequence of reduction of the ability and/or the willingness to do daily duties, restriction of social contact;
(4) use of family or professional help and remedies.

Somebody is ill who perceives an impairment of his sense of well-being and who labels this state as illness, who disengages himself from daily duties because of feeling ill or who fulfils them only partially, who stays off from work because of a decline in the willingness to work (in this case, illness may be the individual's strategy to relieve himself of the overload on his job), who uses medicaments or folk remedies, who uses other family members or a nurse for help, who contacts a doctor or who lets himself be hospitalized.

For the same person, these indications may occur separately or be combined, each with different manifest actions. Some variables can be determined only subjectively (for example, anxiety, pain, fatigue, uneasiness), some objectively (for example, functional disability, use of help). But all can be measured in a standardized way, for example in an interview survey.

In medical sociology, the relation between the characteristics of a person in a specific life situation and his behavioural reaction to perceived signs of illness, given his attitude, available information and knowledge, is called *illness behaviour* (Mechanic 1968). Different types of persons react very differently to the same subjectively perceived phenomena. Socioeconomic and situative (enabling) as well as psychosocial factors (status specific symptom awareness, health consciousness, etc.) are important variables in this context (Siegrist 1977).

Parsons (1951) has conceptualized the main aspects of illness behaviour in the sick role, which according to him involves:

(1) exemption from normal social responsibilities;
(2) the sick person not being expected to get well by an act of decision or will, that is he is exempted from responsibility for his condition;
(3) the sick person wanting to get well;
(4) the sick person co-operatively seeking technically competent help.

The starting-point of Parsons' definition of the sick role is that the concept of health relates not only to the individual but also to the society to which the individual belongs. Health for Parsons is '. . . the state of optimum capacity of an individual for the effective performance of the roles and tasks for which he has been socialised'. It is a characteristic of a healthy society that the incidence of sickness remains small, so that the overall productive capacity remains high. Because the incidence of sickness is mainly controlled by doctors, who professionally define somebody to be healthy or sick, the health delivery system must ensure that individuals do not enter the sick role too early. On the other hand, starting the sick role too late has disadvantages too, because the individual may need sick status in order to recover quickly and to regain his role in society.

To measure the state of illness (health) of individuals and groups of people on the basis of the above items, the following components may be useful:

(1) number of days with complaints with or without restrictions of usual daily activities. Complaints and impairments of normal behaviour can be further differentiated in different states of perceived illness;
(2) medicaments used with or without prescription, or other remedies used for therapeutic purposes;
(3) number of contacts with physicians, subdivided into specialities, and other ambulatory health personnel;
(4) number of days confined to bed at home or in an institution.

To quantify the state of health of groups of people on the basis of individual data, the percentage of individuals with specific states within each group may be used.

Approaches to the assigning of values to different states within one component, perhaps on an interval scale, and to describe the state of health by single or multidimensional health indices, are described elsewhere in this book (see chapter 3).

Illness from the Physician's Viewpoint

From the viewpoint of the physician somebody is ill who visits him in his practice with a suspected illness, or who belongs to his list of longterm patients because of a chronic disease which has to be controlled. For this group of persons the sick role is identical with the patient role. Usually the doctor determines a reason for consultation which he notes as 'diagnosis'. In so doing he relies on the patient's complaints, which he ascertains during the consultation, and on diagnostic data, which yield positive or negative findings. Even when the findings are negative, he will write down a diagnosis to justify his claim on the public insurance plan (as in the FRG).

Although they lay claim to medical scientific validity, these 'diagnoses' can be classified only under relatively broad categories of diseases known in medical science. Fine differentiation is not possible due to the limited diagnostic and therapeutic skills of the physician.

In cases of complaints without diagnostic findings, for example in psychological disease, a classification into scientifically clear categories is even more difficult, because here the doctor relies completely on the statements of the individual and, in terms of time and education, does not have the capacities of a specialist like a psychiatrist. As a consequence, the use of words by the doctor to describe disease is idiosyncratic and variable (Von Feber 1978).

Many patients with chronic diseases and even severe conditions have no, or only minor, manifest symptoms and do not suffer from any impairment. This may be due to the nature of the disease, to self-conditioning by the patient or to the medical treatment he regularly receives. In such cases, the doctor is the only source for a judgement about health or illness, whether on the occasion of a visit for a preventive check-up or an acute health problem. For these cases, the 'submerged iceberg' of illness in the population is very large.

Another reason for contacting a doctor may be to obtain medical expertise, for example, to determine the relation between a physical, mental or social disability and some putative causal congenital malfunction, injury, or disease. Such authoritative assessments are often required by law to justify specific claims of the patient on social security. In the Federal Republic of Germany, for example, doctors have to confirm any inability to work so that wage payments are not interrupted. General practitioners have an important social control function in determining those objective medical indications and subjective complaints of the patient that may justify absence from work. In other cases of financial benefit from sickness, where abuse is possible, many health systems require medical certification.

The data collection system corresponding to this view of sickness will be characterized by:

(1) kind and number of diagnoses;
(2) kind and volume of diagnostic and therapeutic services;
(3) kind and number of prescribed medicaments and therapeutic services outside the doctor's practice;
(4) transfer to specialists for diagnostic and/or therapeutic consultation;
(5) transfer to hospitals for inpatient care and treatment.

Using these data to grade patients in terms of severity of illness, and to describe the morbidity spectrum of a region by aggregating the data, would be a difficult, if not impossible task. Only rough categories could be derived, requiring the assumption, for example, that patients who are transferred to hospital are, on average (and with the exemption of certain cases such as maternity cases), more severely ill than others. The variance between doctors in the treatment of specific cases is presumably too great to allow for inter-doctoral aggregation and comparison. Characteristics of the doctor (for example, medical specialty, age, medical schools visited, years of practical experience) and the health system (for example, insurance system, doctor's fee system, number of doctors per region, doctor/ population ratio) are, among others, important complicating factors.

To draw a valid picture of the health status of a region on the basis of the medical data of its individuals, a specially arranged data collection scheme is necessary. One example of this kind is the US Health Examination Survey (National Center for Health Statistics 1965).

The Medical-Scientific Concept of Illness

From the viewpoint of medical science somebody is ill whose physical or mental functioning deviates from some postulated norm so as to create personal and/or social problems for himself and/or the community. If the data show findings in accordance with a disease model, his case can be classified according to diagnostic categories. The value of the diagnostic process lies in the fact that determining a specific disease theoretically implies aetiology, prognosis, an appropriate mode of treatment and care. Although for many − not most − diseases the aetiology is as yet unknown or only incompletely confirmed, the symptoms may describe the disease condition so that a specific treatment is indicated. Other disease models are well-confirmed but no effective treatment is known.

Thus, the overall effectiveness of scientifically oriented medical practice depends on (Mechanic 1968):

(1) the advancement of scientific knowledge about particular aspects of biological functioning, as described in a specific disease model;
(2) the availability of diagnostic techniques and the ability of the doctors correctly to identify symptom complexes;
(3) the advancement of scientific knowledge and technical abilities to develop effective remedial measures.

Scientifically oriented medical practice normally implies hospitalization: the validation of findings determining a specific disease is often possible only by longer observation and thorough examination, which both require specialized medical knowledge and technical equipment.

Beyond a differentiation according to diagnostic categories, for example, using the International Classification of Diseases (ICD), patients can be further classified in terms of:

(1) number and kind of further diagnoses beyond the main diagnosis (including complications);
(2) operations;
(3) need for medical and nursing care;
(4) length of stay.

By using the ICD, cases are classified only on a nominal scale; but specific diseases can − by medical judgement regarding, for example, chances of treatment, recovery, age, specific numbers of sick days, expected years free from disability — be graded in different severity classes to give an ordinal scale. The above-mentioned characteristics can be included in such a judgement of severity, too. To measure different needs for medical and nursing care, interval and ratio scales (for example, in money terms) can be developed, referring to the average use or another norm as the standard by which greater or lesser needs are identified. (Interval and ratio scales are defined and discussed in chapter 3.)

Illness from the Viewpoint of Preventive Medicine

In addition to curative medicine, embodying a concern for the detection and treatment of clinically manifest symptoms and complaints of individuals, specific health programmes have been introduced in many countries to detect early or presymptomatic stages of certain diseases. For a comprehensive health prevention programme, however, these steps are not sufficient. Some therefore advocate starting prevention not only at the early stages of illness, but already at the behavioural level of the clinically still healthy individual. From this viewpoint, somebody is at risk (or potentially ill) who exposes his health to known and as such confirmed risk factors: cigarette smoking, overeating, lack of physical exercise, abuse of alcohol, medicaments and drugs.

It may be questioned whether an extension of the concept of illness to potential illness can be limited to the behaviour of the individual in isolation. This does not harmonize with the theory that illness is the result of an interaction between man and his environment. According to this concept (Thienhaus-Grotjahn 1978), factors that determine the origin and the pathogenesis of illness can be divided into those that depend

(1) only on the individual (age, sex, hereditary factors);
(2) on the individual and his environment (immunity, nutritional state, behaviour patterns, social class);
(3) on the physico-chemical environment (climate, air pollution, housing, working place);
(4) on the biological environment (viruses, bacteria, animals, plants);
(5) on the psychosocial environment (family, society, school, job situation).

This means that, in preventing illnesses, both the individual and his environment have to be considered. As far as psychosocial factors are concerned, these can be divided into

(1) those that describe specific life situations and which might have a stressful effect on the individual (that is a biologically definable reaction of the organism to specific environmental stressors);
(2) those that describe specific socially influenced behavioural patterns or attitudes of the individual, which might lead to stress reactions and biological malfunction (for example, the so-called type-A-behaviour pattern, which is presumed to be a cofactor in the pathogenesis of cardiovascular diseases. (Dembrowsky *et al.* 1978);
(3) the specific manner or situation or ability of the individual to cope with stressful life events.

A variety of scales have been developed to measure the severity and cumulative effects of stressful life events, specific behaviour patterns and coping abilities. Siegrist *et al.* (1980) in a retrospective study comparing former patients with heart attacks and matched controls, constructed a global index of the interval type. This index combined several subindices measuring chronic and acute stress situations of the individual before the incidence of the disease and the effect of different coping capacities. The higher the global index before the outset of the disease the larger the differences in ratios between cases and controls.

The Framingham (Truett *et al.* 1967) and other studies have shown that morbidity and mortality rates of specific subgroups correlate highly with the number of risk factors including psychosocial factors in these groups and also with the severity scores obtained. It can be shown that the risk of reducing life expectancy by specific life styles can be predicted using multilog-regression functions with the number and value of specific risk factors as independent variables. Thus, for the development of a comprehensive indicator system to describe the health status of the population, risk factors like smoking, drinking, overweight, drug abuse., etc., and other factors which lie in the environment of a person, should be collected.

CONCEPTS OF HEALTH

There is a widespread agreement that health is more than the absence of illness. Health has a positive dimension. Constituent elements are well-being, efficiency, willingness to work, energy reserves to get along with the requirements of the environment or, as Parsons (1951) defines it, the capacity and functional fitness for the performance of approved social roles.

Health is a state of balance between man and his environment and is a prerequisite of self fulfillment (Thienhaus-Grotjahn 1978). This state is not static, but must be re-established continuously as man interacts with his environment. Along with this goes a continuous mutual adaptation. In so far as a state can be reached in which a person can fulfil his life and considers himself to enjoy physical, mental, and social well-being, he is healthy.

V. Ferber (1978) emphasizes the danger of stressful environment and therefore defines health as a state in a process of mutual adaptation that must meet two criteria:

(1) guarantee physical functioning (circulation, respiration, metabolism, digestion, motion, sensation), also for a conceivable future;
(2) guarantee of an unrestricted participation at the age-, sex-, and class specific socialization process, also for a conceivable future.

This guarantee includes the right to the protection of the individual's health from the environment. The demands placed by society on the individual should not be such as to endanger his health defined as above.

This approach is closely connected with the more comprehensive concept of the quality of life for which, in several research projects, many indicators have been developed. Here health is but one of a large number of factors (Berg 1975 pp. 3—22, Zapf *et al.* 1977).

By analogy with the concept of risk factors, restitutional factors (Schaefer *et al.* 1978) may also be considered in health indicator system. These factors describe those influences on health that counterbalance the effects of risk factors or mitigate them. As with risk factors, these factors originate from the psychosocial environment (for example, enjoyment, satisfaction, appreciation, recreation), from the technical environment (for example, parks, noise protection measures), or from individual behaviour (for example, physical activities, 'moderation in all things').

3

Issues of Measurement in the Design of Health Indicators: a Review

RACHEL ROSSER[1]

INTRODUCTION

The design of a heaith status indicator is commonly seen as a two-stage process.

Description

States are defined by descriptions and thus a nominal scale is constructed. The definitions may be detailed and potentially infinite in number (see for example Torrance); limited to a circumscribed, but relatively large, number (for example Bergner); systematic and fairly comprehensive, but fewer in number (for example Rosser and Watts); systematic but limited to particular groups of patients (for example Katz); or systematic with claims to being a comprehensive and fundamental classification with content validity (Bush). The merits and properties of different classifications or sets of descriptions remain controversial and the choice is partly determined by the applications of the indicator, and partly by the type of scale envisaged.

Scaling

Descriptions are placed, often by psychometric methods, on an ordinal, interval, or ratio scale. The requisite level of measurement depends on the intended applications of the indicator. A wide variety of methods have been used to elicit these scales, but the properties of the resulting scales remain contentious.

[1] I acknowledge with gratitude the help of Paul Kind, whose reading and thinking particularly influenced my discussion on the meaning of measurement.

This review traces the development of the measurement of illness for health indicators. It is written in the following sections:

(1) the meaning of measurement;
(2) a historical review of the literature on health indicators;
(3) a selection from earlier reviews.

THE MEANING OF MEASUREMENT

Theory of Measurement: Definition and Classification

Definition. Modern theories of measurement can be traced back to the work of Russell (1920) and Stevens (1946), although there is also a nineteenth century literature which bridges the disciplines of philosophy and physics. These early investigators conceived of measurement as an assignment of numbers or numerals either to objects or events (Stevens), or to properties of objects (Russell, Campbell, 1920) according to a set of rules (Torgersen, 1958). The rules might change but the entity being measured remained the same. However, Dingle (1950), discussing the impact of the theory of relativity on the theory of measurement, argued that quantities do not exist but are imputed by the operation of measurement. He defined measurement as 'any precisely specified operation that yields a number'.

Campbell's Classification. Campbell's classification of types of measurement was based on the empirical procedures used to measure physical phenomena. Two forms of measurement were defined: *fundamental*, which does not rely on the measurement of other magnitudes (for example length) and *derived* (for example density) (Campbell 1920). However, with appropriate instruments, it is possible to proceed directly to the measurement of so-called 'derived' values. Ellis (1966) has therefore suggested that Campbell's classification is more accurately labelled *direct* and *indirect*.

Stevens' Classification. Stevens' classification (1946) has had a major influence on the development of measurement theory. It defines a hierarchy of four types of scale representing different levels of measurement. The first and second are qualitative measures based on the process of sorting, of which ordering is a special case. The first, a nominal scale, is a synonym for 'description' or 'labelling'.

A set of definitions, a list of names or a classification, involves *nominal* measurement. The second, an *ordinal* scale, involves ordering the measured entities in terms of one or more properties, for example weight, intensity, beauty. The other two are both quantitative or *cardinal* scales and thus constitute true measurement. The third, an *interval* scale, defines the distances between ordered entities, for example temperature in degrees Fahrenheit. The fourth, a *ratio* scale, defines both distance and proportion and has a true zero, for example weight in kilograms. It falls at the top of the hierarchy and embraces characteristics of all other scale types. Hence a ratio scale can be used, not only to determine ratios between two points on a continuum, but also to describe the relationship between two points in an ordinal sense, that is in terms of algebraic inequality. Whilst Stevens himself saw the possibility of extending the number of scale types by including, for example the logarithmic interval scale, he suggested that his classification was fairly exhaustive in practical terms. Coombs (1950) followed Stevens' approach but introduced a number of other types and included scales which lie between, for example, interval and ordinal scales.

Scaling Techniques

Level of measurement. Different techniques *aim* to produce scales of different types but investigation of the level of measurement *actually* achieved and the relationship between scales produced by different methods has only recently been undertaken.

Psychophysical techniques are often based on the untested assumption that subjects can and do perform the specified numerical operation, however difficult this may be. Techniques based on confusion or discrimination between stimuli may be the least intellectually demanding.

Comparative judgement. Thurstone's method of paired comparisons (1927) was the first successful attempt to translate some of the experiences in measuring perception of physical continua into the measurement of attitudes or values. His scaling technique makes no assumptions about the inherent scaling abilities of a subject. Subjects are only asked to compare pairs of entities and to state which of the pair possesses more of a chosen property. Thurstone provided systematic theoretical support for his technique founded on the assumption that the degree of inconsistency between subjects scaling such comparisons is monotonically related to the real psychological distance between the entities.

Ratio, partition and confusion scales. Stevens also made the transition from measurement of physical continua to the measurement of opinion and other moral and aesthetic variables. However, the theoretical basis for his psychometric techniques has never been adequately expounded. He advocated the use of a modified power function to describe the relationship between perceived magnitude and the physical value of the stimulus. For the most part, he used methods that require subjects to make direct estimations of the magnitude. These procedures belong to a class of operations known as cross-modality matching. A typical experiment employing this technique would involve subjects matching numbers with apparent lengths. The subjects might then be asked to produce lines which matched loudness or brightness. When loudness and brightness were matched with numbers they produced essentially similar functions (Stevens 1964).

Matching judgements that involve the use of number are particularly prone to bias and error. An individual may be potentially capable of arithmetic operations involving a range of numbers but, in practice, his own experience may limit his performance. Stevens noted that perceptions of number and length have been shown to be almost linearly related and suggested an initial exercise involving matching numbers and lines as a means of initiating subjects into more complex uses of number.

The techniques used for scaling attitudes and opinions have been extended to include the cross-modality approach of Stevens. For example Dawson and Mirando (1976) investigated the ease and difficulty of pronunciation of groups of three letters using a dynamometer.

Stevens distinguished between two types of continua: *prothetic* (quantitative) and *metathetic* (qualitative). Partition scaling techniques require the subject to partition entities that actually fall on a continuum. Category scaling, using a scale of equal appearing intervals, is a special case of this. When partition techniques are used on metathetic continua, the resulting scale is linearly related to a magnitude scale for the same continuum. In general, prothetic continua produce a concave curvilinear relationship between the two scale types (Stevens, J C *et al.* 1960, Stevens, S.S. 1960). This indicates that subjects do not in practice use the intervals as equal. The relationship may become linear if the logarithms of the magnitudes are used.

These terms may appear obscure, but the distinction must be made between types of continua when an attempt is made to establish the level of measurement actually achieved by a particular scale (see for example Patrick *et al*. 1973b and Kind and Rosser 1980a).

The relationship between interval and ratio scales produced by these methods has been investigated by experiments on non-physical attributes. Stevens (1966) summarized many of these studies. They include occupational preference, aesthetic value of handwriting, music, and seriousness of offences. Both Sellin and Wolfgang (1964) and Ekman (1962) have studied the seriousness of crime, although Ekman's study was principally methodological. In this study, pairs of statements about criminal or immoral behaviour were given to subjects, who were asked to indicate the worse statement in each pair. They were then asked to estimate as a percentage how bad the worse statement was compared to the better one. An interval scale was constructed from the paired comparisons, and a ratio scale using the geometric means of scores for each statement. When the two scales were compared, a logarithmic relationship was found. Sellin and Wolfgang used a category rating procedure to produce the interval scale and a direct magnitude estimation procedure to construct a second scale. Once again the relationship between the two scale types was logarithmic. The theoretical background to the relationship between category and magnitude scales has been investigated by Eisler (1962).

A third class of methods additional to magnitude production and partitioning depends on identifying confusion or failure to discriminate between entities on a continuum. These are based on the assumption that equally often noticed differences are equal. This is a special form of the assumption made by Fechner (1907) that just noticeable differences (JNDs) between entities along a continuum can be used as equal units on an interval scale of sensation. For metathetic continua, this assumption can be supported, since the scale based on JNDs is linearly related to that based on magnitudes; but for prothetic continua the relationship is again curvilinear and thus a scale of equal intervals cannot be constructed. The same limitation applied to paired comparisons methods (Stevens 1959a).

Thus the choice of method of constructing a cardinal scale for a new continuum is limited, since the relationship between scales produced by different methods differs for different continua. Stevens therefore argues that it is best to aim from the start for a ratio scale, using methods of magnitude estimation or production.

Psychophysics is not without its critics. Luce (1972) holds the view that psychophysical measurement is not related to physical measurement. He does not dismiss the work of Stevens however, but suggests that the impressive results obtained from magnitude estimation and other procedures should act as an incentive to the development of measurement theories that can explain these results. Savage (1970) goes further in denying that sensation can be measured or related to stimuli. Stevens dismisses this view as a philosophical one which is not open to rebuttal. Luce's appraisal of psychophysics is however more reasonable. He sees the experimental subject as a measuring device. This 'device' receives many physical inputs and psychophysics seeks to describe the ways in which the input is coded and processed by the 'device'. The same coding mechanism may not operate when a subject is asked to perform two different scaling procedures.

Applications: their relevance to choice of scale for use in health services

For the purpose of comparative evaluation, phrased in questions of the form 'How does the outcome of intervention A compare with the outcome of B?' a nominal scale may be sufficient (for example 'died or survived'), but an ordinal scale is likely to provide greater statistical efficiency because a smaller sample may answer the question if a more sensitive measure, such as an ordinal scale of severity, is used.

When the question is phrased in the form 'How much more effective is A than B?' a cardinal measure is needed and at least an interval scale is required. If the question is phrased in the form 'proportionately how much better is A than B' or 'What resources should we allocate to A and B?' a ratio scale is preferable.

In choosing a scale, one must take into account the uses which *should* be made of it, and those which are *likely* to be made of it. A ratio scale is open to less misuse than an interval scale, but if a scale is incorrectly claimed to have ratio properties, it may be used inappropriately in informing decisions.

Associated with each scale type is a class of permissible transformations between measures x and y. These are (i) linear transformations (interval scale) of the form $y = ax + b$; (ii) positive scalar transformations (ratio scale) of the form $y = ax$. The difference between these two classes seems on the face of it, relatively trivial, merely the existence of a 'true' zero. However, the existence of this property may prove difficult to establish, and an error in assuming its existence may lead to important misinterpretations of data and hence to erroneous decisions.

The Concept of Utility

In the following discussion, the term 'utility' is used synonymously with 'subjective valuation' as applied to states of health of illness. This term is used with greater or lesser precision, by writers on economics, psychophysics and decision theory, to mean the value assigned to money or to commodities. The theory of utility is complex and owes much to the work of von-Neumann and Morgenstern (1947) who devised the technique of the standard gamble. Using this technique, subjects are asked to choose between a *gamble* with a desirable outcome with risk p and a less desirable outcome with risk $1-p$, and a *certain* option of intermediate desirability. The method yields an interval scale. Thurstone (1931) also approached the measurement of utility indirectly by plotting indifference curves, a method in which the subject reports how much of a commodity bundle A he needs to be as satisfied as he is by standard amounts of a commodity bundle B.

For Stevens, the concept of utility provided the bridge between the measurement of perception of physical stimuli and the valuation of moral and asethetic concepts (Stevens 1959a). As for physical stimuli, he advocated direct measurement of utility on a ratio scale. However, he indicated that little was known about the relationships between the results of direct and indirect methods and, at present, the choice of method may be determined by the intended applications of the results (Hull, Moore and Thomas 1973).

HISTORICAL REVIEW OF HEALTH INDICATORS

In this section, no distinction is made between the terms 'indicator' and 'index'. Measures are reviewed that claim to be direct assessments of a population's health, and that consider either morbidity, graded by severity, or both mortality and morbidity; measures solely of mortality or of disease prevalence are thus excluded. Measures that are applicable to all or most age and social groups and to all or most specialities and diseases are reviewed comprehensively; those that have more limited applications are reviewed only if their originators conceived them as special cases of a more general measure, or if their methodology has since been seen to have wider implications. Consequently, many measures designed for use solely in clinical decisions or controlled trials are excluded, particularly if they are restricted to particular diseases or specialities. Also excluded are perceptual social indicators, which measure people's sense of well-being or happiness, but are not specifically related to health. These were reviewed by Abrams (1976).

The Concept of Combined Indicators: the Phase of Description or Nominal Measurement

One of the earliest contributions was Stourman and Falk's review of the usefulness of existing statistics as indicators of the state of health of populations (1936). They concluded that combining indicators to produce a single index would be of little interest and might result in loss of information of relevance to individual problems. Nevertheless, interest in such combinations increases.

Logan and Brooke (1957) described the background and results of the Survey of Sickness, 1943 to 1952. They defined its objective as the provision of a three monthly index of morbidity. The proposal for such an index was made by the General Register Office as a means of investigating the impression that, despite falls in conventional indicators, (for example maternal and infant mortality rates; proportion of stillbirths; standardized mortality rates; and prevalence of infectious diseases) complaints of minor ailments and general ill-health were increasing. The index would supplement statistics on trends in public opinion and habits collected by the wartime Social Survey. It would take into account deaths from non-violent causes and serious, moderate and minor illness, and ill-defined symptoms. The authors traced the history of such enquiries in Britain, starting with the Report of the Poor Law Commissioners in 1838. They reviewed many more recent surveys of the prevalence of specific diseases and of disability and impairment, but concluded that there was no single existing source from which a complete picture of the nation's sickness experience could be gained. The situation was similar in other countries.

Painstaking attention was paid to data gathering and the authors critically assessed their own results. They calculated the sickness rate (number of people reported to be ill in a month), prevalence rate (number of illnesses), incapacity rate and medical consultation rate. An important contribution of the survey was to identify the large amount of ill-health for which people do not seek treatment. However, Logan and Brooke concluded that sickness rate and prevalence rate were so heavily weighted with minor and trivial illnesses that they were too stable and inert for an index of sickness prevalence. The other two measures, they concluded, suffered from lack of clarity and comprehensiveness. Despite their initial aim to devise an index of sickness, they did not attempt to combine their summary statistics into a single index and suggested that future surveys should focus on more limited and clearly defined issues.

Alternative conclusions are possible. For example, the sensitivity of the statistics might be increased by splitting down some of the categories and defining them more precisely. Furthermore, the changes in attitudes to the Health Services since this survey have led to more concern about minor, untreated illness. It is thus not surprising that other workers were less pessimistic and that there has been increasing worldwide interest in both morbidity surveys and indices of health.

A World Health Organisation Study Group on Measurement of Levels of Health listed prevalence surveys in many countries (WHO 1957) and suggested two classifications of health indicators. In terms of the first, indicators could be: (a) associated with the health status of persons or populations in a given area (for example vital statistics, nutrition) or (b) related to physical environmental conditions with more or less direct bearing on health status (proxy measures) or (c) concerned with health services and activities (for example availability and use of hospitals or doctors). In terms of the second, they could be: (a) *micro*, that is related to an individual or (b) *macro*, that is related to groups. The groups apparently did not discuss whether micro-indicators could be aggregated to provide macro-indicators or vice versa. They listed available statistics such as crude death rate (which they commented was too insensitive to provision of health services) and infant mortality rate. They considered a new index called the proportional mortality ratio defined by Swaroop and Vemura (1957) as the number of deaths at age 50 or less as a proportion of all deaths, but they doubted its validity or applicability. They recommended research on indicators of morbidity, absenteeism, nutrition, mental health and use of health services. No appropriate existing indicators were identified.

Draper (1963), developed some of the ideas of this WHO report and suggested that data from different sources on the prevalence and incidence of disease and the duration and severity of disability should be combined to form indices of preventable and unavoidable infectious disease, of minor malaise, degenerative diseases and diseases due to particular causes such as pollution. These would be supplemented by data on the average length of spells of illness and the number of attacks per affected individual. However, no major conceptual developments emerged directly from either the WHO report or Draper's paper, and the ideas were not converted into operational measures.

The Concept of Scaled Descriptions

In contrast, several groups of researchers in the next two decades adopted an entirely new approach to measuring levels of health. All these proposed measures had in common the idea of defining the states of patients in a standardized manner and placing scores on these states to represent their relative positions on a scale of severity and to permit them to be combined. Proposals differed in their comprehensiveness and in the scoring systems used.

Indices of Activities of Daily Living: the Phase of Ordinal Measurement

Katz *et al.* (1963) outlined the Index of Activities of Daily Living (ADL) designed to describe, for clinical purposes, the states of elderly patients. Patients were graded on ordinal scales of ability in bathing, dressing, transferring, toileting, continence and feeding. Scores on individual scales were summed, all scales being treated as equally important, thus yielding a single total score. On the basis of more than 2,000 evaluations of states of patients, the authors observed that these functions were lost in order and that the process of recovery resembled child development. They therefore claimed to have a measure of fundamental biological as well as psychosocial function, a claim that has since been questioned by workers using Guttman scales (for example Williams *et al.* 1976). The index of ADL was shown to predict the long-term course and social adapt-ation of patients with strokes and hip-fractures and was used to evaluate outpatient treatment for rheumatoid arthritis (Katz *et al.* 1964, 1966, 1968 and 1970).

This group later developed a survey instrument for obtaining health status data containing questions about the need for and use of health services and attitudes towards medical care. Five categories of 'need' were defined and ranked: no disability, restricted activity with no chronic conditions, restricted activity with chronic condition, mobility limitation and bed disability. These were chosen to permit comparisons with existing national surveys. Use of services was also categorized but no method of combining these data was suggested (Katz *et al.* 1973).

In 1964, Wylie and White reported nine years of experience using the Maryland Disability Index which, like the Katz index, gave scores to activities of daily living and was intended for assessment of chronic care. Five, ten or fifteen points were assigned to differing degrees of performance in each activity, yielding a maximum score of 100. The score was assigned jointly by a physical therapist and a psychiatrist in discussion with nurses and other doctors. However, the focus of this assessment was the extent to which each activity, when regained, reduced the need for nursing care. Thus the measure was designed primarily to reflect need for nursing care rather than health status, and had more in common with measures of nursing dependency, which are based on work study concepts, than with indices of health status. Despite this, there is evidence for the validity of the index as a measure of health status. In a sample of nearly 500 patients with strokes and an index score below 60, the score was predictive of mortality. In another sample of 359 patients, change in score correlated with an independent classification of outcome as 'unchanged' or 'improved'.

The Katz and Maryland Indices were two of the earliest and most extensively tested of a group of indices for use in evaluating geriatric and chronic care. These and twelve others were compared in a review by Skinner and Yett (see below). As they are not comprehensive in application, their details fall outside the scope of this review.

Sanders (1964) made the important observation that improved health care may, by promoting survival of the old and of the disease-prone young, result in an increase in the prevalence of chronic disease. Hence traditional indices of health service performance such as infant mortality rates and standardized death rates may show improvement despite rising morbidity. Furthermore, he argued that health could not be considered as a directly observable characteristic; to measure health it was necessary to choose between a variety of 'potentially measurable characteristics'. He proposed that the effectiveness of health services be measured by their contribution to the increase in economically productive man years. This answers the objection to mortality measures but restricts his measure to the working population and, despite his criticisms of other measures, it does not acknowledge the complexity of the measurement of health.

Maddox (1964) used self-assessment of elderly subjects. He worked with a team at Duke University that devised a system for rating physical and mental health, social and economic resources and activities of daily living on 6-point ordinal scales, that were later reduced to 2-points ('probably adequate' and 'probably inadequate') permitting 32 combinations. The relative importance or severity of the different combinations was not scaled however, and death could not be incorporated into the measure but was added as an extra state. The classification was applied to a sample of 1,000 elderly people in Durham County and found to be predictive of the type of care these subjects were already receiving. This was considered to be evidence for its validity. Sixty per cent of this sample were found to have no impairment as defined by the classification. The authors did not comment on the relevance of this finding to the sensitivity of the measure. The system has also been used in several studies of the cost and use of health services (Maddox 1964, 1972; Burton *et al.* 1978), although it has not been incorporated into a specific mathematical model.

Comprehensive Indices

The next developments led to proposals for more comprehensive measures. Chiang (1965, 1973 and 1976) worked on the mathematical theory of combining measures of morbidity and mortality and his approach was taken further by Chen (1973, 1975, 1976a). Sullivan (1966, 1971) explored the conceptual and practical difficulties and thus laid the foundations for much empirical work, some of which, such as Miller's Q index (1970), also incorporated mathematical formulations of the type that interested Chiang.

One of Chiang's basic equations for an annual index of health was:

$$H_x = 1 - (\bar{I}_x + \tfrac{1}{2}m_x) \quad \text{(Chiang 1965)}$$

where H_x is the mean duration of health per year for a particular age group, $\bar{I}_x$ is a vector representing the effect of states of illness and m_x is the effect of death, derived from available age-specific mortality rates. $\bar{I}_x$ is calculated from $\bar{N}_x . \bar{T}_x$ where $\bar{N}_x$ is the observed average number of illnesses per person per year.

The index H, the weighted average of the mean duration of health per year of the population's age group, is calculated from values of H_x, for each group.

This index was oversimplistic in assuming that days of illness are of equal importance whatever their cause and that death is equivalent to the loss of half a year as a consequence of any illness. It also assumed that time can be handled linearly and that episodes of illness are additive, whatever the characteristics of the individuals afflicted and whether or not the episodes are recurring in the same individual or affecting different people. These latter two assumptions are common to many indices and are discussed by various reviewers such as Torrance (1973 and 1976).

With the benefit of thinking by other researchers, Chiang introduced a further equation to take into account severity (Chiang 1973, Chiang and Cohen 1973):

$$H_x = \sum_{i=1}^{S} w_i e_i$$

where S_i is the state of health of the ith individual, w_i is the weighting given to S_i on a scale of severity and e_i is the fraction of a year spent in S_i.

In the later paper (1976), he reviewed work done by others since 1965 on description and scalings of states and incorporated some of their ideas. He now expressed the index as a matrix of which the elements were the expected incidence and duration of states and the probability of transitions between each state.

Sullivan (1966), in a practical, concise and influential review, discarded clinical and subjective criteria of ill-health in favour of more readily observable and quantifiable behavioural criteria. He first suggested an index constructed from a set of states of impairment of performance in social roles, expressed on a scale indicating their relative importance. Later (1971) he envisaged three indices; the conventional expectation of life, expectation of disability-free life and expectation of life free of bed disability. Using published survey data, he estimated these for the USA in the mid 1960s as 70, 65 and 68 years. These figures are of interest because more recent workers have claimed there is a larger gap between crude and disability-free life expectancy, thus arguing more strongly for the need for health indicators.

A third development was made by the Centro de Estudios de Desarrolo and the Pan-American Health Organisation (concepts in Ahumada *et al.* 1965, formula given in Fanshel and Bush 1969). Their formula was designed for use in developing countries, where reduction of mortality may still be the major objective of health services. It compares the priority P, or relative importance, of a disease by:

$$P = MIV/C$$

where M is the ratio of the incidence of deaths due to the disease and all deaths; I is the product of the number of deaths from the disease and an age-dependent coefficient; V is the vulnerability of the disease to health service intervention. MIV is thus an effectiveness index and P, being related to costs, is a cost-effectiveness ratio. The idea of including V is important, but it is difficult to estimate in practice. Later workers have therefore not developed it. I, which weights individuals according to their economic productivity, might not be universally accepted, and it is arguable that the inclusion of M and I leads to double-counting.

Many of the indices proposed in the next decade had features in common with one or more of the three measures described above.

Magdelaine *et al.* (1967) discussed methods of describing the states of patients so that they could be scaled to form an index. They dismissed diagnostic classifications as too complex and distinguished two principal criteria, the risk of death and the effect of the illness on the life of the individual. To these they added the probable course of the illness. Using these criteria, they defined seven stages ranging from absence of illness to a fatal illness. They then defined the states of a population of 2,820 males by a two stage process: a screening interview, supplemented, if possible, by medical information. They did not, however, move beyond an ordinal scale of the importance of the states and thus the application of the measure would be restricted to evaluation.

Proxy Measures: the Indirect Approach

At this point, a digression from the mainstream development of direct measures of ill-health was made by Kische *et al.* (1969). They sought a brief, objective measure which would correlate with judgements that might be made by clinicians and would yield a cumulative mathematical score. They devised an interview containing questions about admissions to hospitals, medication, and acute and chronic conditions during the previous year. Scores were assigned on the basis of duration of medication and type of disease or symptom. These were summed with certain exclusion rates, to yield a proxy health status score (P). In two studies of 188 and 87 patients, statistically significant agreement was obtained between P scores and grading of patient's health by clinicians as good, medium or poor, although P scores were biased towards a more optimistic assessment of health. All questions were not of equal discriminative value, the question about hospital admission being of least use. This index used arbitrary scales of arbitrarily chosen criteria and there was no justification for their aggregation. In scaling it added nothing to earlier work. Its descriptions of states resembled those used in the wartime sickness survey, but they were less clearly defined. Not surprisingly, the approach was not fruitful, but it has been described here because comparable proxy measures are still proposed from time to time (for example Spautz 1972; Levine and Yett 1973; Allison 1976; Hightower 1977).

Miller (1970) also used surrogates of morbidity in his Q index. This was designed for the assignment of priorities in the Indian Health Service and had features in common with the Pan-American P index. He used degrees of loss of productivity as the basis for value judgements about states of dysfunction and death. He assumed the following values:

(1) a day as a hospital in-patient is equivalent to a day lost by premature death;
(2) a day spent as an out-patient is equivalent to a third of a day lost as an in-patient or by death;
(3) everyone up to the age of 15 is assigned a potential of 50 years' productivity;
(4) everyone over 65 is assigned a potential of half a year's productivity;
(5) diseases are weighted by a factor which gives priority to those that affect Indians most relative to the national average.

No justification was offered for these values, nor for the potential impact of the emphasis on productivity in planning care for the elderly:
The equation is:

$$Q = MDP + \frac{274A}{N} + \frac{91B}{N} + \frac{274C}{N}$$

where: M is the health problem ratio (target group: reference rate)
D is the crude target group mortality rate per 100,000
P is years of life lost due to premature death from disease
A is number of in-patient days
B is number of out-patient days
C is days of restricted activity
N is target group population

274 is a conversion constant $(\frac{100,000}{365})$

91 is a conversion constant $(\frac{274}{3})$

These arbitrary assumptions might possibly be acceptable for an index to aid planning in a primitive society, but would have to be modified for more advanced cultures. However, the Q index is unusual in that, whether or not it is appropriate, it has been used routinely for planning a health service.

The Phase of Cardinal Measurement

The approaches set out so far suddenly gained new impetus with proposals for indices applicable to more advanced cultures from groups of researchers, under Bush in the USA, Card in Glasgow. Torrance in Canada, Culyer and Williams in York and Rosser and Watts in London. Packer (1968) in an isolated theoretical paper, had defined seven states ranging from absence of disability to death, but suggested the need for cardinal measurement. He drew on the economic concept of utility, or value, and thus proposed a scale which would not only order states of illness, but quantify the extent to which they were perceived as undesirable.

The Work of Bush's Group (San Diego)

General approach. Fanshel and Bush (1970) reviewed and structured the field in what has become a classic paper. They conceptualized 'severity of illness' as a composite of dysfunction and prognosis. Eleven functional states were defined, ranging from complete well-being, a theoretical state, to death. The severity of these states would be scaled. An arbitrary upper limit to human life was set at 90 years (later extended to 100 years, Bush *et al.* 1971). The prognosis of a group of individuals in any state was conceptualized as a function of their probability of moving from this to every other state. People at death entered a reservoir for a series of finite time periods until reaching the age of 100. This formulation is in terms of a stochastic process represented by a stationary Markov chain. This is a standard Operational Research Model and many properties automatically follow and the permissible mathematical transformations are known.

The approach is theoretically elegant; the problems lie in converting it into a practically useful instrument. These were anticipated in this paper and some were tackled in a group of later publications (Fanshel

1972; Chen and Bush 1971; Bush, Fanshel and Chen, 1972; Patrick, Bush and Chen 1972 a and b; Bush, Chen, and Patrick 1973; Blischke, Bush and Kaplan 1975; Chen, Bush and Patrick 1975; Chen, Bush and Zaremba 1975; Kaplan, Bush and Berry 1976; Bush, Kaplan and Berry 1977). Most of the work has focused on the description of scaling of states of patients; their studies of applications have been limited and very little attention has been given to prognosis.

Description. States of health were defined as 29 likely combinations of four levels of capacity for physical activity, five levels of mobility and five levels of social activity. These were combined with 42 symptom and problem complexes (Patrick *et al.* 1973 a and b). It was claimed that this system provided a set of jointly exhaustive and mutually exclusive states, derived from a search of survey instruments and medical textbooks, only mental health problems being excluded.

There seems, however, to be no justification nor need for this claim of exhaustiveness. Indeed in a later paper (Kaplan *et al.* 1976), 14 further function levels were defined, as a result of experiences of classifying patients, and there are no obvious grounds for precluding further levels and even further dimensions of ill-health. Basic properties, especially reliability, had not been tested, and the choice of 42 symptom/problem complexes was clearly arbitrary, the possibilities being virtually limitless.

Scaling. Three psychometric methods, all self-administered in booklets, were used to show that the relative severity of these states could be scaled. The first was category scaling. Subjects rated each state on a scale of 15 equal appearing intervals, on which death had been assigned a score of zero and optimum function a score of 16. Judges were asked to rate the desirability of a day in each state, each judge considering 200 descriptions of states of health occurring in people of five age groups. A marked 'truncation' effect was observed, judges tending to choose scores towards the centre of the scale. When the states were ranked, the scores assigned to about three quarters of them were statistically significantly different from those assigned to adjacent states. The judges were either nurses or graduate students and the former gave consistently higher ratings ($p < 0.02$) although statistical correlation between the scores of the two groups was high ($r = 0.91$). (However, since the scores for some of the states were skewed, parametric statistics were not strictly permissible.) The authors acknowledged that the crucial test of the significance of differences in the scores produced by different judges would be the sensitivity of data on patients or populations to the application of different scale scores. They also suspected that judgements were contaminated by judges' guesses about the prognoses of the state.

In a second experiment, two groups of students and 'health leaders' rated 50 descriptions chosen because, in the earlier study, they yielded low inter-rater variance. In addition to category ratings, they used methods of equivalence and magnitude estimation. Whereas it was possible that category scaling might yield only an ordinal scale, the other methods were expected to yield cardinal measurements, and probably ratio scales.

The equivalence method aimed to identify the judge's point of indifference between keeping alive a group of people in a 'standard state' of perfect health and a larger group, of a size to be defined by the judge, of less well people. This was treated as the most self-evidently valid of the methods, having the best theoretical foundation in classical psychophysics, and was thus the criterion against which the other methods were validated.

The method of magnitude estimation assigned a score of 1,000 to a day spent by a person in a state of perfect health and the judge was asked to choose a score between 0 and 1,000 to represent the proportionate desirability of a day spent in each of the other 50 states.

These three methods are well-established in psychophysics and derive from the work of Stevens (Stevens 1959) on the perception of physical stimuli such as sound and the measurement of judgement or value (Stevens 1966). The work of Patrick *et al.* was derivative from that of Sellin and Wolfgang (1963) who applied psychometric methods to the valuation of crime seriousness.

Certain limitations in the methods are obvious. Firstly, the method of equivalence was phrased ambiguously and some subjects might have found it morally unacceptable. Secondly, in classical ratio scaling, it is usual to set only one end of the scale during the experiment, although the other end may be arbitrarily defined to standardize the measurements when analysing the results. Thirdly, time is assumed to be perceived linearly in magnitude estimation. Fourthly, it is assumed that severity is perceived independently of the number of days spent in a state. Separate experiments would be necessary to investigate the legitimacy of these assumptions.

Patrick *et al.* studied the reliability of their methods. Test-retest reliability with a limited number of repeated items was modest (r ranged from 0.74 to 0.83 but, as noted above, may not be an appropriate statistic). Statistically significant ($p < 0.01$) agreement was obtained between all three scales from both judges, r ranging from 0.60 to 0.79, but the method of equivalence was found to cause problems of comprehension. In view of the correlation and the apparently linear relationship between category and magnitude methods, some comment on the level of measurement obtained seems necessary, but the authors did not offer this until later, when a curvilinear relationship was obtained by using an 'unbounded magnitude method' (Bush *et al.* 1977). If the scales were to be accepted as ratio, they would rate such states as being confined to bed for a day in a special care unit with an amputation as only four times as severe as states of minimal social disability, such as might be caused by an upper respiratory infection: such scores would be unconvincingly out of line with medical practice and other social behaviour. The range of the magnitude scale was particularly small and the group eventually advocated the use of an interval scale derived by the category method, (Kaplan, Bush and Berry 1979). They also commented on some of the problems of category scaling (Blischke *et al.* 1975). They argued that the 'truncation' effect was due in part to the existence of states 'worse than death' and 'better than health' as they had defined it, thus casting doubt on their claim to comprehensiveness. They also noted that, although the intervals appeared equal, they were used by judges as if they were wider at the ends. They corrected for this by using a fourth degree regression model, by which they obtained a close fit between observed and expected equal interval data both with 'perfect health' set at 1 and death at 0 and vice versa.

At this stage, using a new nomenclature, they claimed that their point of time Index of Well-Being was ready for use. They noted that they had been unable to define the concept of prognosis operationally, but still aimed to use the concept of transitional probabilities. They therefore intended to reduce the number of function levels to a much smaller set and to develop statistical methods to estimate 'function level expectancies'. They would use data from samples obtainable in health interview surveys and from a series of such samples, they would generate 'synthetic cohorts'.

These statements reflect a major change since 1971 (Chen and Bush 1971) when they had planned to use a method of measuring group opinion, the so-called Delphi technique (Dalkey 1969a and b), to obtain estimates of transitional probabilities from groups of experts, and had claimed success in obtaining such estimates for phenylketonuria (Bush *et al.* 1973). It would not have been feasible

to repeat this experiment for all diagnoses, nor would it be so easy
with less thoroughly defined and researched conditions; the contribution of factors other than diagnosis in determining prognosis
(Querido, 1963) would also complicate matters. In two other papers
in 1975, (Chen, Bush and Zaremba 1975; Chen, Bush and Patrick,
1975) other authors were criticized for defining too few states of ill-
health and thus producing crude measures. It is not clear whether a
more sensitive 'point-in-time' measure, and a separate, less sensitive,
index including prognosis were now envisaged. Some revision of
earlier opinions about sensitivity may have been prompted by the
discovery that some of the states were assigned identical psychometric values (Bush, personal communication 1980).

Validity. The group summarized their theoretical work in their most
far-reaching paper since 1970 (Kaplan *et al.* 1976), in which they
discussed the concept of validity in relation to their Index of Well-
Being (formerly called the Function Status Index). They argued that
criterion validation, usually the most conclusive procedure, was
impossible in the case of a health index, as there was no existing
measure of proven validity to use as a criterion. They therefore
adduced a variety of less conclusive evidence. They claimed that they
had achieved *content validity* because the items (descriptors of states
of ill-health) adequately represented the domain they were supposed
to measure, and exhaustively covered the full range of possible states
from perfect health to death. They reported that they and other
workers had classified the degree of well-being of more than 10,000
people, including a study in 1974 and 1975 of more than 1,000
households in San Diego. Their index showed change in both acute
and chronic illness, which they adduced as further evidence of
content validity.

In addition to content validity, they considered the *convergent*
or *construct* and *discriminant validity* of the Index of Well-Being.
The evidence for convergent validity, which depends on consistency
between the experimental measure and several similar or related
measures, was as follows:

(1) people known to have a larger number of chronic diseases were
     assigned lower scores by the Index of Well-Being than people
     with fewer conditions;
(2) people with more symptoms received lower scores;
(3) people who consulted doctors more received lower scores;
(4) people who were independently selected from their sample as

'dysfunctional' received lower scores than the rest of the sample;

(5) older people received lower scores;
(6) the correlation between self-rated health on a 10-point scale and the index score assigned by an observer was positive.

Evidence for discriminant validity, which is established if a series of unrelated and dissimilar measures yield different results from the experimental measure, was as follows:

(1) index scores correlated most highly with self-rated health on the day of assessment and progressively less with self-ratings for the previous seven days;
(2) index scores correlated better with self-ratings of state today than with self-ratings of overall health status, which are presumably contaminated by prognosis.

The appropriateness of the statistics that were used to analyse the data on validity is dubious, since the distributions of the data were not presented and parametric statistics were applied throughout. However, the overall weakness of the evidence seems more crucial. This paper usefully defined the problems of validating such measures, since it is true, as with any innovatory measure, that there is no criterion against which they can be validated. Nevertheless, disregarding the tenuous claims for content validity, the claims for construct and discriminant validity are unconvincing. The evidence does little more than show that the index is not totally invalid. What is needed is a series of measures of related concepts of similar sensitivity to that claimed for the Index of Well-Being, for it is not surprising that the index was found to be generally consistent with such crude indicators. The need for criterion validation seems inescapable and it will therefore eventually be necessary to apply such an index to a series of diagnostically homogeneous groups simultaneously with other measures of outcome of proven validity. This will be a laborious, costly and lengthy process and does not seem to be worthwhile until greater confidence can be placed in the descriptions and scale of states of illness.

Applications. This prolific research group has made one other contribution by applying their index. The original health status index (Fanshel and Bush 1970) was modified and applied to a tuberculosis prevention and treatment programme in New York. Five function states were defined and the probabilities of transitions between states were estimated on the basis of discussions with staff and reviews of the literature. It was impossible to obtain data sufficient to justify a Markov Chain analysis, but the authors concluded that the contribution of the programme to 'dysfunction-free-years' was small and the possibility of ending it was considered. Such a decision would seem premature, given the primitive state of the instrument.

The second application was to phenylketonuria. Eleven experts on the disease met for a day and defined fifteen states of dysfunction. The experts scaled these by magnitude scaling. Graduate students re-scaled them by category rating. There were discrepancies in ranking between the two scales and some obviously illogical orderings. The range of the magnitude scale was 0.083 to 1.0 (both ends being pre-determined) and that of the category scale 0.343 to 1.0. Thus the ratios represented by the scales are 1 to 13 and 1 to 3. The shapes of the scales (the increments between states) were also very different. The authors did not discuss these discrepancies, but preferred both the magnitude method, since it ought to yield ratios, and the experts, since they ought to know. These experts then assessed transitional probabilities by the Delphi method. Data from screening programmes on states of patients and services were used to calculate a cost-output ratio. The estimated output in terms of dysfunction-free-years was found to be independent of choice of scale. No inference was made from this, but it seems to suggest that devoting much effort to accurate scaling may not be worthwhile.

In a paper by Kaplan *et al.* (1976) on validity, the application of the FSI to a household survey was reported. They made the important observation that the gap between traditional life expectancy and weighted life expectancy was 12 years. This, in contrast with Sullivan's study, suggests that health indicators may give a picture of health of the population that differs substantially from that provided by available statistics.

Reynolds *et al.* (1974) claimed to have used the Function Status Index in a survey of two counties in Alabama. However, they made crucial modifications. Social activity was subdivided into role activity and self-care activity, increasing the dimensions of the index to five. Five states along each dimension were ranked in severity and the resulting ordinal scores were summed without regard to the relative importance of the components. No attempt was made to use any of the scales in Patrick *et al.* They claimed construct validity as the index scores correlated weakly with age, use of health services, self-rating of health and self-rating of worry about health. These authors seemed to have missed the point of much of Bush's group's work. One valuable contribution, however, was their emphasis on the distinction between health related dysfunction and dysfunction due to other causes.

The Work of Torrance (Hamilton)

General approach. Torrance's work resembled Bush's in defining a set of states of ill-health and scaling these, but differed in the absence of a classification, its lesser emphasis on prognosis, its choice of scaling methods and its emphasis on use of a health index in planning models (Torrance 1970; Torrance *et al.* 1971 a and b). Torrance defined the aim of a health service as 'the maximization of health index units within specified constraints'. (He at first used the term 'index' to mean the utility or value which society attached to a day in a particular state, but later resorted to its more general usage.) He explored two techniques for measuring utility and two algorithms for the optimum allocation of resources within health services. He introduced the important concept of discounting the value of future health to the present and argued that the utility of a state would depend on its duration.

Description. His psychometric experiments were based on standard descriptions, called scenarios, of a typical day in the life of a patient with a kidney transplant, on home dialysis, on hospital dialysis, confined to home by illness or confined to a sanatorium. States of perfect health and death were used to define the ends of scale. Despite the inclusion of an epidemiologist, Torrance's group did not explain how they chose the features descriptive of a 'typical' day. Their 'worked examples' included studies of the cost-effectiveness of screening for rhesus disease of the newborn and for tuberculosis, a coronary emergency service and a renal dialysis and transplantation programme. The possibility of increasing the sensitivity of the method by definition of more states was not explored. Thus, in contrast with Bush's group, which searched for a comprehensive and valid classification, this group assumed such an approach to be unnecessary and chose to scale an arbitrary set of clearly defined states.

Scaling. In the first study of Torrance's group, eleven general practitioners, acting as judges, scaled five scenarios by two methods. The first was a form of the von Neumann-Morgenstern gamble. Judges were first offered a choice of remaining health for time t, then either being in a defined poorer health state (represented by a 'scenario') for time t, followed by death, or receiving a drug which had a probability p of ensuring health for time t followed by death, and a probability $1-p$ of causing immediate death. The judge had to choose the probability p at which he would be indifferent between the two choices. He then had to make similar choices using each of the other scenarios, but for subsequent choices the reference state was not death, but the first scenario. This method has the advantage of sound foundations in utility theory (von Neumann and Morgenstern 1947). It has two major disadvantages; firstly it is very difficult to understand and thus can only be used with intelligent judges (who nonetheless tend to produce highly variable responses) and secondly, it may measure risk aversion as well as judgements about health. A minor and modifiable disadvantage is that, in the form used here, it tended to assume that death was the worst possible state. This would be unacceptable for the valuation of states of extreme suffering.

In the second method, called time trade-off, judges chose between being in a state defined by a scenario for time t, followed by death, or remaining well for x, a shorter time than t, and then dying. The indifference point was obtained by varying x. This method was easier, but had the disadvantage of assuming that time was perceived in a linear way, that the relationship between the utilities of the states remained constant with time and that no changes in ranking of the states occurred as their duration increased. For example, for a short period, some people might choose the convenience of hospital dialysis; for a longer period, they would probably want to be at home. The experiment, phrased in days, might not detect this, and the tacit assumptions that linearity and constant ranking were self-evident might deter judges from objecting. Torrance himself later showed the limitations of this assumption. 'Disguised' scenarios were used to examine test-retest reliability which was considered satisfactory. The risk of changing the content by means of the disguise was taken because the authors though that valuations might be too unstable to permit delayed replication. The entire interview lasted up to 45 minutes.

Mean utilities ranged from 0.34 for sanatorium confinement to 0.83 for a kidney transplant. In a later paper (Torrance *et al.* 1973), full results were published, showing that the utilities assigned to each state were very variable. For example, the utility assigned to sanatorium confinement varied from 0 (that is at least as undesirable as death) to 1.00 (as desirable as perfect health!). The distributions of the results were not characterized, but they were analysed by parametric statistics. The coefficient of correlation between the two scales was 0.95, the mean difference between the paired values was not statistically significant, and the scales were therefore assumed to be equivalent.

As a detailed demonstration, the utilities for four scenarios were applied to data from six tuberculosis screening programmes and their cost-effectiveness ratios were calculated. These programmes were also compared with renal and haemolytic disease programmes and large differences in cost-effectiveness were shown. However, the crucial test of the method, the sensitivity of the conclusions from data about patients to scales of utility derived by different methods from different individuals, was not undertaken. Haemolytic disease programmes were later compared with 11 other screening and treatment programmes (Torrance and Zipursky, 1977).

Torrance then increased the number of scenarios to 15 (Torrance 1976; Sackett and Torrance 1978), including states due to mastectomy for carcinoma, chest surgery and depression. He now moved away from the restriction of a single day and performed three separate experiments for states lasting three months, eight years and for life. These were scaled by his previous two methods and by a category method with a 10 cm visual analogue scale. Test-retest studies were done for the first two methods using disguised scenarios, but although the correlation coefficients were reasonable, there was evidence that the 'disguise' changed the content of the scenarios in some important way and thus the degree of reliability remained elusive. Three groups acted as judges, a stratified sample of the population of Hamilton, Ontario (*N=246*), 29 patients on renal dialysis and 43 graduates of McMaster University. Only the graduate group performed the standard gamble and even for them, it was made easier by the use of a coloured probability wheel. (The likely effect of such a technical modification on the results was not discussed.) The precise disease 'label' mentioned in the scenarios somewhat affected the results.

All methods were found acceptable and feasible. The category method was quicker and easier; its reliability was not reported but Torrance's impression was that it was not satisfactory. The full results have not yet been published but, again, parametric statistics were used throughout without comments on the distributions of the results. The time trade-off method was described as a variant of magnitude estimation. In contrast with Bush's findings, the relationship between the results of this method (T) and of category scaling (C) were not linear but described by a modified power function:

$$C = 1 - (I - T)^{.62}$$

This reportedly gave adequate predictions of the mean utilities from groups but not from individuals. Presumably therefore, inter-individual variation in this experiment was high.

Torrance used the standard gamble as a criterion against which to validate the other methods, presumably because of its theoretical soundness. He concluded that the time trade-off was valid ($r = 0.98$ for population means and 0.65 for individuals) and the category method less so ($r = 0.81$ for populations and 0.36 for individuals). The low correlations between individual results from the two techniques highlight the contribution of technical artefact and the importance of ensuring the subject understands the exercise. The importance of discrepancies in the results for health service applications was not discussed. Some trends and some statistically significant differences were found between scales from subjects of different age, sex, socioeconomic group and health status. Women, for example, preferred dialysis whereas men preferred transplantation; older subjects tended to be more accepting of in-patient treatments.

The Work of Card's Group (Glasgow)

Card has also focused mainly on the measurement of the utilities of states of illness and, in addition, on the valuation of life (Card and Good, 1970). Like Torrance, Card used standardized descriptions of states of illness, and made no attempt to derive a classification. However, whereas Torrance worked within the framework of planning models, Card's motivation for estimating utilities was to incorporate them into decision models with the aim of formalizing clinical decisions. He noted the very high variability of the valuation of life implicit in various social decisions (Card and Mooney, 1977) but used mock decision situations to obtain highly invariant estimates of utilities from clinicians.

He studied gastro-intestinal diseases to which specialists assigned severity weightings expressed as percentages. For proctocolitis, he identified several dimensions of severity, performed a number of ranking exercises, and then, using a method which has not been described in detail, he transformed the ordinal results into cardinal ones using standard mathematical tables. He also considered the utilities of states of head injury. He anticipated that utilities would be converted into money equivalents for cost-benefit analysis and to inform resource allocation (Card 1975). He used a wagering method, potentially sensitive to risk aversion, in an elegant experiment on medical and non-medical subjects. They chose whether or not to offer an operation to a patient who might, as a consequence, recover his sight to varying extents or become blind. All impairments of vision were confined to one hypothetical patient and thus the descriptions of states of illness fell along a single, very limited, dimension, but the authors speculated that the method could be extended to multidimensional situations and thus gain more relevance to real medical decisions (Card *et al.* 1977).

The decision theory approach was also advocated by Barnoon and Wolfe (1972) in an approach to the evaluation of the impact on a lifetime's disability of an individual intervention. This had features in common with Chiang's mathematical models (see above) and Culyer *et al.* (1971) (see below). Gustafson and Holloway (1975) developed such concepts in detail in designing and validating an index of the severity of burns using a scaling model known as multi-attribute utility measurement. This scaling approach was also used By Plishkin and Beck (1976) in an index designed to inform clinical decisions about the management of end-stage renal failure. These two papers are mentioned, despite the limited applications of the results, because they differ from others in assuming that ill-health cannot be scaled along a single dimension.

The Work of Culyer, Lavers, Williams and Wright (York)

Culyer, Lavers and Williams (1971, 1972) started with a substantial theoretical paper. Like Card, they anticipated the conversion of utilities into monetary equivalents. They distinguished indicators of three types: state of health (SOH) indicators, that would combine medical data and judgements with social judgements. need for health (NFH) and effectiveness indicators, the latter two being functions of the former. They spelt out the importance of eliminating from SOH indicators (which are the type to which the terms 'index' and 'indicator' most commonly refer) all 'input content' so that the effect on SOH of varying resources could be examined. They envisaged an individual's health as a series of states, comprising combinations of pain and dysfunction of varying duration and terminating in earlier or later death. Such a concept was also used by Chiang in his later work (Chiang 1976). The effectiveness of a medical intervention

could be assessed by its impact on this series of states. Social valuations would be assigned to these states either politically, by a
government 'minister', or by empirical measurement, but if the latter
course were to be chosen, it would be necessary to investigate whether
a consensus existed in society about the appropriate values. This
formulation is similar to that of Fanshel and Bush, and again, the
difficulty arises in obtaining the data.

Williams, like Bush, decided first to construct an index of states
of health. Like Bush, he also defined several dimensions of ill-health,
each divided into several states, but he regarded these as standard
descriptions, not a comprehensive classification. Unlike either Bush
or Torrance, he gave highest priority to showing that it was feasible
to classify patients in these terms, and lower priority to mathematical
algorithms or scaling. However, he expected that a scale of utility
would eventually be obtained and further hoped, like Card, that it
could be converted into money equivalents. Emphasizing the need
for an instrument for routine rather than research use, he embarked
on a study of changes in the states of a large sample of elderly people
to be classified by care-givers at intervals of three months (Williams
1974). Data collection was abandoned at the feasibility stage, because
sufficient participation was not obtained from care-givers. This
experience has cast doubt on the cost-effectiveness of the indicator
approach to health care evaluation, since it suggests that costly
special surveys may be needed to provide the data.

Despite this discouraging start, Williams' colleague, Wright, persisted
in exploratory analyses of the pilot data (Wright, 1974, 1978).
Performance was graded in four categories along three dimensions
which were: mobility, self-care and mental state. Mobility subsumed
various combinations of four activities: self-care covered a further
eight activities and mental state included confusion, depression,
anxiety and loneliness. Some combinations were ruled out as impossible, for example a person using a wheelchair was assumed to
be unable to climb stairs. Wright, unlike many of his predecessors,
who worked with sets of ordinal scales, was concerned that simple
addition of ordinal ratings might lead to anomalies and to an insensitive index. Many combinations of dysfunction, for example, could
be assigned the same overall score. Furthermore, he found, when
the classification was applied to the pilot sample ($N=360$), a high
correlation between mobility and self-care. He therefore decided to
merge these two dimensions to form a revised ordering for measuring dependency. This resembled that used by Katz in his index of
ADL, and had features in common with the Guttman scale of R.

Williams *et al.* (1976) (see below). Wright also used a three month follow-up of 289 of these pilot study subjects to demonstrate the crucial point that inferences about the percentage change in state were subject to the method used to scale the states; hence the choice of scale was of great practical importance.

The Work of Rosser, Watts and Kind (London)

General approach. This group has focused particularly on indicators of hospital performance (Rosser and Watts 1971, 1972; Rosser 1974; Rosser and Benson 1978; Benson 1978) but also defined the relationship between their measure of hospital output and measures for use in communities and at higher administrative levels (Rosser 1975; Rosser and Watts 1977, 1978). From the start, they obtained the active involvement of clinicians, but have consistently advocated circumspection in their writings for clinicians (Rosser 1981) and planners (Bevan *et al.* 1980). Like the York group, they distinguished between observed loss of function and mobility and subjective suffering and defined 29 combinations of disability and distress. These categories were reliably used by doctors and nurses. They made no claims for the comprehensiveness or the fundamental validity of the system, arguing that what is needed is a standard set of descriptions which can be used reliably and which might be substantially modified in the light of the experiences of scaling and of use in studies of hospitals. They are currently engaged on such an exercise of modification, the aim being to remove redundancies and evaluate more than 70 other constructs, including 'prognosis' and 'duration of illness' with a view to including some of them in a more elaborate descriptive system.

Two principal scales of valuation of these states have been derived by psychometric and behavioural analyses. The psychometric scale (Rosser and Kind 1978) was obtained from 70 subjects with different personal experience of illness, including medical and psychiatric patients, medical and psychiatric nurses, hospital doctors from various specialities, and health volunteers. Fifty other subjects took part in a reliability study. The method was based on the principles of magnitude estimation, but used a lengthy and elaborate individual interview procedure devised by Gibbs and Wishlade (see below) in their work on crime seriousness. The features of the interview included a detailed discussion with the subjects of the context in which their valuations were being elicited and the uses of the resulting indicator, much attention to the subjects' ability to work with ratios, and time for discussion at each stage of doubts, changes of mind and causes of confusion.

The range of the resulting scale (1 to 500) was very much greater than those obtained by Bush *et al.* and by Torrance's method, but was not out of line with current practices of resource allocation. Methods of fractionation and multiplication were also used to provide some evidence for the internal validity of the scale. Furthermore, when the data were processed as a paired comparisons exercise, the resulting interval scale X could be transformed into a ratio scale Y with a close fit ($r = 0.93$, $p < 0.001$) to the empirical ratio scale Y by application of the appropriate theoretical predictive equation for a prothetic continuum which is:

$$log_e (Y) = aX + b$$
$$(Y) = e^{aX + b} \quad \text{(Kind and Rosser, 1980a)}$$

This provides strong support for the claim that the subjects were producing ratios at interview.

The other scale was obtained by the analysis of legal awards for the non-pecuniary consequences of personal injury and industrial accidents and disease (Rosser and Watts 1975). This method had the major disadvantage that many factors must contribute to the precise amount of the award in addition to the assessment of the severity of the injury. Judges, however, have often claimed that a scale of appropriate awards is emerging, and the variance in the scale obtained in this way was no greater than that usually obtained by psychometric techniques. This limitation is offset by the advantage that what people say they feel and would do, may differ from what they actually seem to feel and do. The legal awards scale thus differs from all other scales to date in reflecting actual behaviours and also in being inferred from an existing resource allocation process. It correlated highly with the psychometric scale ($r = 0.81$, $p < 0.001$). For the purpose of further comparison, the two scales were arbitrarily standardized on a 0 to 1 scale with death set at zero and 'not ill' set at 1. This highlighted the relatively high value placed on the more severe states by the psychometric scale, and raised questions of relevance to legal and insurance practitioners. (Kind, Rosser and Williams, 1981.)

The indicator was used in two hospital studies. In the first (Rosser and Watts 1972, Rosser 1975), states of all patients in a district general hospital were categorized by their doctors on admission and discharge and on the first and last day of a one-month study. In the second (Kind and Rosser 1980b), doctors categorized all patients on medical and psychiatric wards for three months, and some patients were also categorized daily by nurses to give a more sensitive measure of the day by day process of care. In these studies, the method was shown to be feasible and reliable, and sensitive to known differences between units and specialities. However, it is also notable that the rankings of different units by output were sensitive to the differences between scales derived from different sources of data (psychometric and legal) or by different statistical analyses (for example different measures of central tendency) of data from the same source, even though the correlation between all the scales was highly significant ($p < 0.001$) (Rosser 1980). This observation is important, since all other groups have accepted statistically significant correlation between scales as sufficient evidence for their validity; too little attention has so far been paid to the validation of scales in application. This problem may be less important in *community* measures than in *hospital* measures but it is not yet clear whether scales of morbidity are much more useful than crude mortality data for community evaluation.

A further contribution has been on the valuation of death (Kind and Rosser 1979). Like Bush and Torrance, the group is still working on feasible methods of handling prognosis, but differs from the other groups in taking issue with previously published scales, many of which implicitly assumed that death was the worst possible state, and assigned to it a value of zero. Two scales were elicited, one for permanent and one for transient states. These were virtually identical except that death was included on the scale of permanent states. Its valuation was highly variable, but its median or geometric mean scale score was lower (that is less undesirable) than those assigned to permanent unconsciousness and to lifelong confinement to bed in severe distress. This is not merely an academic curiosity, since a false zero invalidates any inferences made on the basis of either interval or ratio scales.

The Work of Recent Groups

Since 1971, numerous researchers have worked along similar lines to these five groups, whilst others designed detailed health profiles for community evaluative studies.

Belloc *et al.* (1971) proposed a limited set, say eight, mutually exclusive and jointly exhaustive states, ranging from perfect health, through stages of physical disability, to death. Their original contribution was the use of Ridit (Relative to an Identified Distribution) analysis (Bross 1959). The mean ridit for a population of defined characteristics is calculated from the frequency distribution of states; other populations can then be compared with it (it is not clear why a special label is needed for such an ordinary procedure as comparing two distributions!). In a survey of Almeda County, California, gradients of health were found to be related to sex, age, income and race. Breslow later extended the states to include eight categories of mental and four of social health, which were not combined. The aim was to quantify the World Health Organisation's definition of health. Ridit analysis was used to quantify the extent to which an individual deviated from the population mean. This approach was not pursued by its authors, but in 1972 a group in Taiwan did a survey of physical health in the adult residents of ten cities and, by ridit analysis, confirmed the existence of gradients by age, sex and income (Young *et al.* 1974).

Grogono and Woodgate (1971) defined the following ten aspects of health: work, recreation, physical suffering, mental suffering, communication, sleep, dependency, feeding, excretion and sexual activity. The grounds for choosing these were not stated. All were treated as equally important, and patients were assigned a score on each criterion of *1* (normal), *½* (impaired) or *0* (incapacitated). Scores were then summed. Twenty-seven patients were categorized by 20 medical or student observers. Test-retest and inter-observer reliability yielded correlation coefficients in excess of 0.8. The choice of statistic was not discussed; presumably therefore parametric statistics were used without regard to the distribution of scores and to the inherently ordinal nature of the scales, a score of ½ covering a wide range of impairment. It is not clear whether the patients were inpatients or outpatients, but the authors suggested that the scores be added over time to produce a health index expressed in 'health-years'. They foresaw their instruments being used for a wide range of purposes, from the evaluation of a medical intervention in an individual patient, to allocating resources in communities to treatments and to research. However, they paid no attention to the level of measurement they had achieved and did not discuss their method in the light of previous literature. Hence, the range of applications they envisaged was perhaps over-ambitious.

These authors collected no further data, but Coles *et al.* (1976) compared the reliability of their index with those of Fanshel and Bush, and Rosser and Watts, all applied to the same 32 patients. Reliability was not achieved, but this was not a particularly helpful observation since all the conditions essential for obtaining agreement were disregarded (Rosser 1977).

Grogono's and Woodgate's index was compared with Linn's Rapid Disability Rating Scale (Linn 1967, 1977) in a study of 1079 elderly people by Jenicek *et al.* (1977). Both measures showed a gradient of ill-health with age, but both were criticized as containing insufficient detail for research surveys.

A similar criticism of the health indicator approach was made by Starfield (1973, 1974), who like Grogono and Woodgate, did not place valuations on the relative importance of different aspects of ill-health. Her reason for rejecting valuations, that they would change over time and from place to place, seems insufficient, since most researchers have assumed that scales of severity would need constant updating and could not automatically be translated to different cultures. She proposed that the outcome of medical care should be assessed by a profile resembling the Minnesota Multiphasic Personality Inventory (MMPI) (Dahlstrom and Welsh 1960). By implication, she would sum the ratings of a patient's state along a large number of constructs. Such an instrument would presumably be used for evaluative purposes in a research setting, but by analogy with the MMPI, problems in interpreting the meaning of the constructs might be anticipated. A profile approach has been used by Sackett's group and placed on a firmer theoretical base by Bergner's group, who differ from Starfield in emphasizing the need for cardinal scaling (see below).

A number of researchers made a brief appearance in press as a consequence of a conference on Health Status Indexes in October 1972 (Berg 1973). New data and ideas, which were sparse, are summarized below.

Levine and Yett reverted to the idea of proxy measures of health status (see Kisch above). They chose various socio-economic indicators such as proportion of the population with higher education, owner-occupiers, car-owners, etc. There was no evidence that the index was relevant to health services. Berditt and Williamson described a function limitation scale, for measuring the quality of ambulatory care. Patients were assigned, on the basis of information gleaned on the telephone by a 'health accountant', to one of five ranked functional states. Its construction was primitive and no claims were made for its general applicability. Skinner and Yett reviewed 14 published indices of activities of daily living, including the Maryland Index and those of Katz and of Linn (see above), of which four were designed to yield a single severity score. They advocated the use of Guttman scaling (see Wright above and R Williams below) to assign patients to a dependency class. However, 33.5 per cent of patients could not be accurately assigned in this way. Despite the purely ordinal nature of their data, they claimed they could be related to costs.

Scaling was discussed extensively at this conference. Berg described a study of the utility of 'various conditions' judged by medical students and physicians who performed two exercises. The first was a form of the von Neumann-Morgenstern standard gamble, the choice being between confinement to bed or an operation with a variable probability of restoration to health or death. The second was an equivalence experiment to determine the subject's point of indifference between saving the life of one working man on the top floor of a burning house or a number, to be estimated, of quadriplegics on the ground floor. This second method was obviously contaminated by judgements of such irrelevancies as ease of access to different floors. Both methods resulted in very high variance. Despite the exploratory nature of the work, the author was not deterred from publishing the results. Females, older people and Protestants seemed to be more tolerant of life confined to bed; males showed less risk aversion yet women placed more emphasis on saving the working man (on the first floor!). More systematic studies by other workers have not revealed such personal preference.

Acton tried to deduce the utility of myocardial infarction from what people claimed they would pay for a preventive service. Students made three decisions about investment in a mobile coronary care unit which would reduce the risk of death from a myocardial infarction to the community and to themselves. They seemed to understand the question, but the results were correlated with the income of the subject. Forst described a method of obtaining 'conditional utilities' from individuals. Variables which might affect the utility of a state of illness, for example its duration, painfulness, consequent financial loss and prognosis, would be identified and maps of indifference between combinations of these would be obtained. The utilities assessed by this process would be validated against direct ranking and real behaviours such as risk-taking in traffic. The utilities would then be used in clinical decisions. Limitations of the method include its complexity, the variability of behaviours to be used as criteria of validity, the lack of empirical evidence and contamination of an output measure with inputs such as financial loss.

Theoretical Indices

Chen (1973) proposed the G index, the first of a series comparing the health of a target population with that of a 'normative' one. This was a modification of Miller's Q index (see above) for assigning priorities to the treatment of diseases in underprivileged groups. Like the Q index, it compared the impact of the defined disease on the target group with that in a reference population, but unlike Q, it took into account data on morbidity in addition to mortality in the reference population. It made all the same arbitrary assumptions as the Q index and treated all productive years lost as equal. Chen assumed that all necessary data would be available, but this would not be true for diseases which have been eliminated from the reference population. Chen later (Chen 1976a) reduced the number of arbitrary assumptions, and devised two further 'equity indices' called G'_1 expressed in years lost due to illness, and G'_2 expressed as an index on a scale from 0 to 1.

Chen also modified an index devised by Scheffler and Lipscomb (1974). They proposed two indices, H, to measure the physiological and emotional aspects of functional disability and H', to measure the pecuniary aspects. H consisted of five function levels, weighted by utilities derived by the von Neumann-Morgenstern gamble and applied to published survey data. People ill for less than three months were automatically assigned to state 0. The utilities were defined for any disease, but the index applied to particular diseases, a process to which Chen took exception. He criticized several details in the construction of H and replaced H' with modifications called M and F, M being purely descriptive and F being relative to local norms of income (Chen 1975).

Chen added P and P' to his list of comparative indices. They measured mortality rate relative to the level of health of the living in different countries (Chen 1976b). He also devised the K index (Chen 1976c) based on the concept of 'sentinel events' (Rutstein *et al.* 1976). The K index combined measures of incidence and severity of avoidable and undesirable health events. Communities with the lowest rates were used as a standard. The avoidance of idealized concepts of health seems to be Chen's principal contribution to the health indicator field.

Health Profiles

In contrast with the rather sterile manipulation of broad theoretical values described in the paragraph above, groups under Sackett in Hamilton and Bergner in Seattle favoured a detailed and empirical approach.

Sackett's group (Sackett *et al.* 1974; Chambers *et al.* 1976; Sackett *et al.* 1977; Chambers *et al.* 1978) developed a health index questionnaire containing 120 items covering physical, emotional and social function, supplemented by questions on symptoms and smoking. These were selected from available survey instruments. The questions were unambiguous and designed for administration by survey research workers. Positive responses to questions were summed to give scores for each aspect of function. Scores were found, as expected, to be higher in the young, in discharged rather than admitted patients and in those free of chronic disease. This was said to provide evidence of 'biological validity'. A discriminant function analysis was used to determine the ability of each question to predict general practitioners' clinical assessments. The resulting coefficients were used to weight the responses to each of two sets of questions and the score for each individual was then standardized to yield a social and an emotional index score between 0 and 1. The principal use of such an index is in research. For example, its originators used it in a randomized trial of family nurse practitioners.

Bergner's group (Bergner *et al.* 1975, 1976) placed great emphasis on observed rather than inferred data and thus chose to consider behaviour rather than feelings. Aspects of health for inclusion in their sickness impact profile (SIP) were obtained from more than 1100 postal questionnaires completed by patients, healthy people and health service professionals. 312 items were grouped into 14 categories, one of which *did* cover emotions and feelings. After exclusion of duplications, piloting on 246 patients and item analysis, 235 items remained in the longer form and 146 items in a shorter form.

These were scaled firstly by successive intervals analysis of 15 point category ratings as used by Blischke *et al.* (see above), the raters all being health service personnel. High reliability was obtained and the scores for the items were aggregated in several ways. A second scaling experiment using an 11-point scale was completed by a group of 25 health service professionals and by a stratified sample of members of a pre-paid group practice ($N = 173$). The ratings of the two groups of judges correlated highly, but the group practice judges systematically assigned higher scores. (This bias among judges is the opposite to that found by Patrick *et al.*). The most extremely rated items were rescored on a 15-point scale, but a truncation effect remained. It was assumed that high variability in the scores assigned to an item reflected a weakness in the item, which was discarded. Thus this group disregarded the possibility of true disagreement between the judgements of raters and took for granted the existence of a social consensus. They were meticulous about the internal consistency of their scale, but, having noted the absence of an adequate criterion for external validation, they adduced little evidence for its validity (Carter *et al*. 1976). They noted that it discriminated in research surveys, for which it was designed, between sicker and less sick people. Patients' self-ratings were found to correlate higher (r = 0.76) with first year residents' ratings but poorly with those of more experienced doctors (r = 0.33), the discrepancy being greatest for social and psychological aspects of illness. On this basis, it was proposed as an instrument for training doctors (Martini *et al*. 1976). No attempt was made to aggregate the scores for the 14 categories. The SIP has been translated into colloquial English and re-scaled for use in surveys in London (Patrick, personal communication).

Martini and McDowell (1976) planned to use the SIP to evaluate a rehabilitation centre. They modified it in a manner of questionable legitimacy, reducing the items to a total of 82 within only 12 of the 14 categories. They compared modified SIP ratings of 110 patients with doctors' gradings of activities on four point ordinal scales. Predictably, correlations were highest for observable physical activities and lowest for quality of family relationships. They concluded the instrument was not yet ready for use in population studies. This group has recently published a scale for a new instrument (McKenna *et al*. 1981), but re-analysis of their results casts grave doubts on the unidimensionality of some of their data (Kind 1981).

A second conference on Health Indexes in Phoenix in 1976 again stimulated new contributors. These included Ware, who described a 32-item questionnaire to study people's perceptions of their own present and future health and Wan, who used a discriminant function analysis of data on the health status of more than 11,000 adults living at home, to argue that, since socio-medical indicators such as disability were highly predictive of self-assessed health status, health status indices should focus on function.

Recently two new proxy or surrogate measures of health status have been proposed by Allison (1973) and Hightower (1978). The latter is notable for making, on the basis of a factor analysis of data on 55 demographic and health related variables for the counties of Mississipi, the extraordinary claim that the results of the analysis thus quantify health, something 'which has not been achieved before'.

In contrast, R. Williams, *et al*. (1976), in a cautious and thoughtful paper, described the application of Guttman scaling to a rigorously tested classification of disability designed for use in the elderly and chronic sick (Garrad 1972; Garrad and Bennett 1970). They confirmed that disability progresses in regular, cumulative patterns and, unlike Skinner and Yett (see above), obtained high coefficients of reproducibility and scalability. They used it in a community survey and a study of post-operative patients. In view of the ordinal level of measurement yielded by Guttman scaling, they made limited claims for the application of their method and thought it could be useful in assessing individual disadvantage, predicting progress or deterioration and evaluating the outcome of treatment.

Bebbington (1977) compared Guttman scaling with the results of principal component scaling and of additive scaling (as used by Grogono and Woodgate) and obtained high correlations between them. He therefore argued that, for the purpose of obtaining a broad picture of the disabled population, the choice of numerical values was substantially irrelevant, for any scale which was inherently uni-dimensional. This may be so for the limited applications he had in mind, but correlation coefficients offer insufficient evidence: what is needed to support the argument are illustrations of the inferences which might follow from applying the various scales to survey data.

A SELECTION OF REVIEW ARTICLES AND GENERAL PAPERS

While this section was in preparation, a comprehensive review appeared by Goldberg *et al.* (1979). This is the only published paper that attempts to place North American and European developments in perspective. No previous reviews attempted comprehensiveness but a few aimed to structure the field and are mentioned here. These articles fall into four groups, which consider (a) the arguments for combining mortality and morbibity; (b) the classification of health indicators; (c) conceptual and practical difficulties in their development and (d) methods of scaling. Two other issues, the validity of extrapolating classical psychometric techniques to the measurement of judgement, and the practical advantages of the newer indicators over traditional statistics are not sufficiently considered in the literature on health, although they have appeared in writings in other fields, especially crime.

The Issue of Combined Indicators

Moriyama (1968) compared traditional indicators based on mortality with the new measures proposed by Chiang, Sanders and Sullivan and argued for more research on indicators combining mortality and morbidity. Bickner (1969) disagreed. He listed the potential uses of health indicators as: public information; administration, including choice, planning, reviewing, and finance; and medical science. He recommended that indices of mortality and morbidity be kept separate because 'we have no tolerably good technique for reducing these two elements to a common dimension'. He also favoured separation of measures of degenerative and non-degenerative conditions, because of their very different degrees of responsiveness to treatment, and accidental, congenital and other illnesses, because one consequence of combining these was loss of information of importance for planning.

Damiani (1973) reviewed traditional mortality measures and the work of Magdelaine *et al.* and of Chiang on combined indicators. He completely rejected combined indicators for the time being, because they were based on highly controversial assumptions. Bickner (1976) wrote a sceptical review of the work of Chiang and Sullivan and the proxy index of Spautz. He argued that, at their present state of vagueness, exaggerated claims had been made for the usefulness of combined indicators. He thought that it was premature to aim for both a combined index of health status comparable with measures of gross national product, and a measure of positive health rather than of ill-health. Despite his views on the need for limited objectives, he argued strongly for the combination of input and output statistics, based on current theories about causes and effects.

Bickner's statement about the combination of mortality and morbidity remains true since no research group has devised the valid, practical, and comprehensive measure of prognosis that is a necessary prerequisite for combining statistics on present morbidity with statistics on death rates. However, a modest research investment on the valuation of death relative to states of ill-health seems justified, since choices between the prolongation of disablement and earlier death must be made, and it is to be hoped that the difficulties of measuring prognosis will eventually be solved. The measurement of vulnerability to treatment (the term used by Ahumada in 1965) remains unsolved, and attempts to correct for it by means of severity indices (Roemer *et al.* 1968; Duckett and Kristofferson 1978) have not answered Bickner's comments about degenerative disease. Bickners's concept combines input and output measures, restricts the research applications of an index and violates the economic principles outlined by Culyer *et al.* (1971).

Classifications of Indicators

The design of health indicators attracts taxonomists. I shall not suggest a classification of my own, but list below a few examples.

Nishi (1971) writing in the context of planning, reviewed traditional mortality measures, along with Ahumada's P, Chiang's H, Miller's Q and Fanshel and Bush's original health status index. His language was sometimes ambiguous, perhaps because it is a translation from Japanese. His criteria of classification were the following six 'axes', which were clearly labelled but not always lucidly defined: input-output; indirect-direct; superficial-depth; analysis-synthesis; simple-complex; and static-dynamic.

The four measures reviewed were all categorized as complex and static. The HSI, although considered impractical, was the most comprehensive, direct and output orientated and was 'synthetic'.

Miller (1973) used the following six criteria.

(1) Data requirements: How feasible is it to obtain the data specified?
(2) Scalar characteristics: What is the level of measurement and what is the appropriate measure of central tendency?
(3) Common denominality: Is the same characteristic measured for all diseases?
(4) Comprehensiveness and specificity. An indicator can be other disease-specific, or comprehensive, or both.
(5) Age and sex adjustments. Both age and sex adjustments were considered to be desirable.
(6) Utility (usefulness)
     (a) to determine priorities;
     (b) to evaluate;
     (c) to allocate resources.

These activities form a hierarchy requiring progressively higher levels of measurement.

He noted that all the indices he had reviewed were deficient in age and sex adjustment and demanded data from special surveys. Only Bush's index could be used for resource allocation, but in his view, it was neither comprehensive nor specific and did not have common denominality.

Chen and Bryant (1975) proposed a three-dimensional classification as follows: M, a measurement dimension distinguishing between self and observer reports, A, an applicability dimension distinguishing measures applicable to individuals or populations and O, an orientation dimension distinguishing between measures of feelings, symptoms and performance.

Torrance (1976 a, b) was concerned with the similarities rather than the differences between health indices. He brought together the mathematical formulae for 14 indices, all of which, he said, combined mortality and morbidity data, aimed to be general in their application, and defined health as a continuum of instantaneous physical, emotional and social states ranging from perfect health to death. He showed that they had a uniform underlying mathematical model and distinguished three sub-types: a point in time index, a period of time index (obtained by summing discrete states at points in time during the period) and a health expectancy index, which is the only one of the three to readily accommodate death. A further criterion was the distinction between application to populations and to programmes.

Problems of Development

Problems in the development of health indices were reviewed by Goldsmith (1972) and Torrance (1973). Goldsmith saw the most pressing problem as the definition of health. He quoted the WHO concepts of 'well-being' (WHO 1958), Siegerist's concept of 'rhythms' (1941, 1960) and Romano's concept of 'balance' (1950) as three typically abstruse and ambiguous definitions of health. He described the empirical work of Lawton *et al.* (1967), who concluded on the basis of a factor analysis of items from 30 indices of health, that a single concept of health which could be defined operationally would not be found. He listed the following subsidiary problems:

(1) validity must be established against both clinical and social variables. This seems to have been forgotten;
(2) reliable and valid data are expensive. Available data are inadequate. He did not discuss how far it is feasible to cut the cost of data by designing indices which, in Miller's terms, could be readily collected;
(3) there is no agreed definition of the point at which a person becomes ill. He did not discuss how this problem could be circumvented by means of an operational definition of an 'episode' of illness.

Torrance was particularly concerned with the measurement of

value and listed a number of unanswered questions. These are shown in table 3.1, together with my responses to them.

TABLE 3.1 *Measurement of value*

Torrance's comment	My response
1. Who should place values on states of ill-health for a health index?	This is a second order question since it is not yet clear: (a) how to measure values nor to assess differences between observers. (b) whether there are differences or whether there is a broad social consensus about the severity of illness. (c) whether different values can be aggregated or whether they are mutually exclusive.
2. Are there differences in value systems between people of different socio-economic groups?	This is an unresolved issue, but it would be oversimplistic to search for differences by socio-economic group alone. Other personal characteristics may be more highly correlated with value systems.
3. Is utility of a state a function of time in the state?	Torrance's earlier experiments using time trade-off implicitly assumed that the utility of a state was independent of its duration; his more recent work showed that this is not the case.
4. Are values specific to diseases or can more general states be defined and scaled?	This question stems from uncertainty in the period 1971–1973 about whether general states such as those defined by Bush, could be scaled as satisfactorily as disease specific states such as Torrance's 'scenarios'. Subsequent research has shown that they can be.
5. Are measurements of utility valid?	This important question remains unsolved.
6. Is a linear model appropriate? for example is it equally valuable to extend 1 life for 1,000 days or 1,000 lives for 1 day?	This is a crucial, unanswered question.

TABLE 3.1 *Measurement of value* – continued

Torrance's comment	My response
7. Are all people equivalent? for example is a 5 year extension of the life of a 20 year old equivalent in value to the same extension for a 70 year old?	The issue of the impact of characteristics of ill people other than their illness, for example age, occupation, on the utility assigned to their state of health is important. It is not conceptually insuperable, but a set of experiments has not yet been designed and executed to measure it.
8. What is the discount rate for future benefits?	This also needs empirical investigation, but the importance of the question depends on the way in which prognosis is handled in the model underlying any particular index.

Scaling

In this review, I shall not consider such issues of valuation as are based on concepts of economics and on mathematical theory that have been reviewed by, for example, Whitmore, 1973 and 1976; Torrance, 1976b. The most important of these is the question of whether the aggregation of the utilities from individual judges to obtain a group consensus can ever be legitimate (the problem of social choice). Work in this field casts theoretical doubt on whether health indicators can legitimately incorporate the utilities of more than one individual. However, it does not preclude further empirical work on the measurement of individual judges' utilities since it is apparent that in practice, the stringent conditions under which aggregation is invalid (Arrow, 1963) can be relaxed.

The literature is particularly concerned with classifying scaling techniques by the level of measurement achieved (Miller, 1970, see above, Kneppreth *et al.* 1973). There is agreement that it is easier to achieve an ordinal scale (which orders states) than a cardinal scale (which measures the relationship between states) and to scale one factor rather than several factors. The level of measurement necessary is specified by the proposed users of the health indicator. For comparative evaluation, ranking is sufficient; for planning and resource allocation, cardinal measurement is needed (Culyer, 1978).

Even ordinal measurement can be difficult. Krischer (1976)

reviewed in detail six indices with specialized applications, including the Cumulative Illness Rating Scale of Linn *et al.* (1968), the Abbreviated Injury Scale recommended by the Committee on Medical Aspects of Automotive Safety (1971), the Comprehensive Injury Scale of the same committee, the Injury Severity Score (Baker *et al.* 1974), the Trauma Index (Kirkpatrick and Youmans, 1971), and the multi-attribute severity scale (Gustafson and Holloway, 1975). He showed that, although these measures aimed for scales of different types, they actually all fell into a class known as 'additive value functions' in which it is only permissible to aggregate rankings along several dimensions if the relative importance of each dimension is known. If additivity of the different dimensions or attributes is taken for granted, the rank-ordering property of the scale is violated. This, he concluded, had occurred with all six measures. He mentioned Plishkin and Beck's work on renal failure (1976) as an example of the correct use of a scaling method (multi-attribute scale) which did not violate this principle.

Culyer (1978) made a similar point in a review of many of the scales already listed in this chapter. He quoted a population study of physical, mental and sensory handicap by Harris *et al.* (1971). In this study, ratio values (that is cardinal numbers) distributed along eight dimensions were added for each individual and the resulting scores were used as rankings (that is to produce an ordinal scale). The authors thus performed an operation that would be valid for combining ratio scores along equally severe dimensions to produce an overall ratio score, but that was invalid for an ordinal scale. One solution to this problem of multidimensional ranking is provided by Guttman scaling as used by Skinner and Yett, R. Williams *et al.* and Wright.

When cardinal measurement is attempted, the problems are greater, because the judge is asked to perform a more difficult task of quantification and there is doubt about the validity of the less difficult methods of attempting this. Alternative methods have been reviewed by Patrick (1976). The theoretically most sound measure, the von Neumann and Morgenstern standard gamble, is difficult to understand and, as previously discussed, may be contaminated by varying risk aversion. Indirect methods of measurement, such as the method of paired comparisons (Thurstone 1927) suggested by Fanshel and Bush (1971) are impractical for more than a few states. Direct estimates, including category scaling (as used by Patrick *et al.* and by Torrance) and equal appearing intervals (as used by Patrick *et al.* and Bergner) are manageable in the laboratory, but would be more difficult to use in larger studies of the valuations of a sample of the population. Patrick concluded that more work was needed on psychometric techniques and on the following questions:

(1) how static are social preferences?
(2) are valuations specific to particular decisions?
(3) how far do valuations depend on the context in which they are elicited, for example on the phrasing of the questions, on the number of states scaled, and so on.

In addition, he advocated more attention to ratio scales of states of health with a zero origin and measurable distances from the origin.

Rippere (1976) reviewed studies of ratio and interval scales of seriousness of illness in the light of related work on the scaling of stressful life events. She compared the results of magnitude estimation with those of direct interval scaling. The magnitude method was used by Holmes and Rahe (1967) to scale life events, and by Wyler *et al.* (1967) to study the seriousness of 126 diseases. Wyler *et al.* chose peptic ulcer to be the 'modulus item' with a score set at 500. Judges could assign to each disease any score above 0 to indicate their judgement of its severity relative to that of the modulus item. The direct interval method was used by Paykel (1974) to scale life events. Judges assigned scores to events on a scale of 20 equal appearing intervals. Rippere applied these methods to the scaling of diseases and found that they were both reliable, gave similar ranges of ratios and correlated highly, but the interval method had the advantages of simplicity, and of yielding less variable and normally distributed results. However, Hough *et al.* (1976), also reviewing the scaling of life events, queried whether Holmes and Rahe's method yielded a true ratio scale.

The numerical results of the work on diseases and on life events is not directly relevant to the subject of the present review. The work is mentioned because important general problems emerge. The questions of obtaining true ratios, and of validity, have not been investigated sufficiently in health applications of psychometric scaling. Correlations between the results of different psychometric techniques such as those reported by Rippere, and of different statistical analyses of results of a single technique, as reported by Masuda and Holmes (1967), have been accepted as evidence of validity. However, Nunally and Durham concluded, in their discussion of measurement in evaluation research, that no scales have intrinsic reality, but are conventions based on agreements between scientists on how to measure (Nunally and Durham, 1975). There-fore, 'strictly speaking, one validates not a measuring instrument, but rather some use to which the instrument is put'. Work on the measurement of crime seriousness has been slightly less deficient in these respects and this review therefore ends with comments on this field.

The extension of psychometric scaling to the valuation of health followed the pioneering work of Sellin and Wolfgang (1964) on crime seriousness. Questions which have been studied in this field and which await investigation in relation to health include:

(1) can apparently minor variations in psychometric technique produce highly significant differences in the resulting scales? (Gibbs 1970, 1972 and 1974);
(2) do scales of valuation, however sophisticated, contribute information which cannot be obtained from simpler, more traditional measures? (Hindelang, 1974; Blumstein 1974; Welford and Wiatrowski, 1975).

SUMMARY AND CONCLUSIONS

The importance of scientific evaluation and informed planning of health services is now widely recognized. In more developed countries, traditional indicators, such as life expectancy and infant mortality rates, may not be sufficiently sensitive for these purposes. A new type of indicator has therefore been proposed which summarizes the morbidity in a community and may combine this with a measure of mortality.

Such indicators define the state of health of a population or target group at a point in time and measure change during a period of time. 'Expectancy' indicators have also been proposed. These measure the expectation of morbidity or combine this with mortality data to form an index of disability-free or healthy years. These indicators share two features: they all include standard descriptions of the states of health of people and a scale which either orders or places cardinal values on the severity of these states. Expectancy indicators include prognosis, but the practical problems of obtaining data on this have not been solved. Indicators differ in their purposes, which range from clinical evaluation to national planning, and in details of their construction.

Differences occur at the descriptive and the scaling stages of measurement. Whereas some indicators aim for a comprehensive classification of states of health or of illness, others aim only for a set of standard descriptions of states and some contain detailed descriptions of 'typical' states, which are not intended to be systematized. The descriptive criteria may be more or less objective, some researchers choosing to sacrifice such important criteria as the subjective experience of illness in favour of clearly objective behaviour, while others maintain that such exclusions place unacceptable limitations on the measure.

Description is the most important stage of measurement, because it may well exclude some aspects of ill-health, which thus receive a zero valuation. However, the most innovatory feature of health indicators is the second phase of measurement — the scaling of valuations — and it is on the methodology of this stage that research is currently focused. For some purposes, such as the comparison of the output of two clinical units, an ordinal measure may be adequate. To answer such questions as 'What proportion of ill-health is relieved by service A compared with service B?' that are necessary in planning resources, a ratio scale may be necessary (such a scale could also be used for evaluation). However, there is still controversy about precisely what type of scale is needed and there seems to be increasing disagreement about the most appropriate scaling technique. Canadian and British workers have favoured methods of magnitude estimation aimed at producing a ratio scale. American workers have recently rejected magnitude estimation in favour of category scaling, which yields, at most, an interval scale. Thus the development of the measurement of the severity of illness is repeating the history of the measurement of crime seriousness. In the field of criminology, opinions remain sharply divided after some 20 years of research; and psychometric scales have so far proved to be of little practical value. After ten years in the field of health services research, scales of illness severity seem likely to meet the same fate unless agreement is reached on the type of scale appropriate to various applications, on methods likely to produce such a scale and on techniques for ascertaining that it has, in fact, been obtained.

Studies of the validity of scales have been limited to measurement of statistical correlation between scales derived by different methods. There is no scale of proven validity to use as a criterion. There is a need for studies of application of cross-diagnostic indices to diagnostically homogeneous groups so that they can be validated against well-established measures of change.

The crucial tests of the validity of scales *in use* have rarely been undertaken. Indeed, all aspects of theoretical development of health indicators are in advance of practice. It has not been firmly established that decisions taken on the basis of health indicators would differ substantially from those informed by mortality statistics alone, and there is a pressing need to apply indicator models to data on people's states of health. Controversy about the methodology of indicator construction thus remains academic, since it is not known whether in general differences in methodology will have practical consequences, although studies by Kind and Rosser suggest that they will do so. Questions also remain about how far people agree on the appropriate scale of utilities, and, if they do not agree, how far and in what way it is legitimate to aggregate different views.

4

Multidimensionality of Health Indicators: the French Discussion

PHILIPPE MOSSÉ

The purpose of this paper is to initiate a discussion of the problem of multidimensionality of health indicators. The paper offers a critical analysis of the French literature, particularly emphasising the problems caused by this aspect of the measurement of health status.

Research workers wanting to classify ill people proceed generally by defining, usually *a priori*, one or several dimensions of health status which are then used to estimate the different levels. The operational definition of the impact of medical care is in almost every case taken to be the difference between health status observed at two different moments. Most methodological disagreements are concerned, on the one hand, with the criteria to be taken into account in the operational definition of health status or, on the other, with ways of measuring the difference between two health states, either for the same individual at two different moments, or for two different populations at the same moment.

Goldberg, for example, writes about the practical problems to be overcome in adopting this approach:

Evidently the first and most important problem to solve is to choose components of an index of comprehensive health status which must be valid and available in realistic conditions especially on the economical level. . . If this stage is realized then another important problem soon arises: is it necessary to introduce a weighting of the different components: and if it is how? Some research workers are against the very principle of weighting. Others, on the contrary, think it is necessary to be able to compare validly situations, either individual or collective, in which health status and the origin of the problems are different. In this case, choices are necessary concerning the different problems: which weighting criterion must be chosen (welfare economics criteria for instance?); who must be asked to determine the utilities (physicians, ill people, possible users of health services, etc. . ?); how is it possible to aggregate validly (and how to do it?) utilities in a period of time and how to determine the rates to apply? (Goldberg 1978).

Thus, the multidimensional character of health which is the basis of 'medical art' becomes an obstacle to the comparability of the difference in health states. The problem of comparability is inevitable when the outcomes of a study cannot be estimated in terms of cost or any other simple numeraire.

In the literature the problem of multidimensionality is divided into two distinct questions:

(1) how is health to be defined in an operational way?
(2) how are the elements coming from this definition to be combined?

The first question has been answered in many different ways according to the field of analysis and the objectives sought. As to the second, it remains unanswered and traditionally lines up the 'technocrats' against the 'democrats'. The former prefer the experts' judgements, the latter prefer to search for the revelation of collective preferences.

In this paper several items from the French literature dealing with these problems from a general or theoretical point of view, will be quoted.

HOW TO DEFINE HEALTH IN AN OPERATIONAL WAY

In an article, published in 1972, Verges locates the problem by asking whether economic science can satisfy the need for social indicators. For Verges PPBS methods reduce the social field to no more than the classic calculating of costs and monetary benefits. From this reduction emerges the notion of a social indicator. The limitations of such economic analysis make necessary the use of other devices than the simple operation of the monetary calculus. However, since the social field differs from the economic, the same operations cannot be used without danger of:

selecting in the social field what is quantifiable . . . for example, aesthetic pleasure is reduced to the number of people visiting a museum, or measures are mixed that cannot be mixed other than by an entirely arbitrary process that deceives only laymen (Verges 1972).

To escape this dilemma the measures used should be directly linked to a theoretical framework. This framework is lacking in the fied of health even more than in the general area of social science. In the latter, utility theory has been used for a long time and is still used now.

Some research workers are trying to show that behaviour in the health field is rational and consists in optimizing health capital (Grossman 1972). As far as I know, the validity of these models has not yet been proved. Moreover, there are no studies of health indicators that use the human capital theory.

Most research is instead located within a broader framework that is *ethical* and is characterized by a belief either in social welfare or utility defined as the combination of many individual welfares or in social welfare, changes in which could be measured by indicators, and which is defined outside of individual welfares, by 'the revelation of a social value showing a moral, philosophical or political consensus'. (Gadreau 1978).

This ethical frame itself seems to be conditioned by the classical economy it refers to. Thus Gadreau continues:

it seems that health is a privileged field where this consensus (concerning the definition of a social preference) is accomplished and consequently it would be illogical for public decisions concerning health to depend upon the revelation of individual preferences the rationality and objectivity of which are rightly questionable'.

This philosophy is the implicit basis of most of the research trying to develop indicators, the different levels of which are estimated by experts who are supposed to represent the social consensus.

By contrast, Goldberg argues plausibly that as far as health is concerned: 'the definition of an index which could be universally accepted is a utopia' (Goldberg 1978). This opinion is shared by Levy:

in the present state of the statistical information which we have, one should not look for a miracle indicator, a trick indicator. The difficulties encountered, both at the level of comprehending the phenomena and at the level of evaluating them, make the formulation of a good synthetic indicator premature (Levy 1974).

Yet perhaps there is no real incompatibility between the search for a general consensus and the manipulation of less ambitious indicators. This information can be considered a descriptive approach of social reality. Hence we get the pragmatic view that 'from the multiplicity of direct applications of specific indicators will emerge a coherent theoretical background' (Carley 1970). So, far from being a preliminary, the conceptual framework of the analysis should be developed from operational studies. This optimistic epistemological view could be accepted if it were permitted by existing studies. But the great majority of research workers are preoccupied with the short-term usefulness of their indicators and fail to make clear the specific assumptions underlying their work.

Jacquet-Lagreze (1979) is convinced that for a decision maker there is no necessity for *a priori* assertion of criteria (for example invalidity, suffering and so on) with regard to global preference (for example health). He advocates an iterative approach associating the decision maker (for example physician, politician) and the researcher. This approach allows for the possibility of the continuous modification of indices and aggregation processes, taking account of earlier results in subsequent revisions. In fact, in most French studies weighting and index combination methods are chosen by the authors themselves without appealing to any consensus, for in France the client of research and the researcher are usually the same person.

HOW TO COMBINE CHARACTERISTICS IN THE DEFINITION OF HEALTH

It is usual to select *a priori* a single indicator according to which the individuals are classified, not taking the other dimensions into account. The advantage of this method is that it avoids the problem of multidimensionality. The assumption, often implicit, is that, according to the perceived explicit objective, the observation of changes in a single parameter is both necessary and sufficient. This attitude is the most frequently adopted in the macro-economy in, for example, measuring the efficiency of a medical care system in terms of its impact on life expectancy. It is also the approach chosen when therapeutical trials are conducted of the efficacy of a medicine on a single biological parameter. This method cannot *a priori* be condemned; it is clear that many projects that started by tackling the problems of multidimensionality directly finished with a unidimensional analysis.

One widely used method consists in drawing up a list of unidimensioned indicators and then aggregating them to make a single overall indicator. Because the main problem is epidemiological, the emphasis is put on the link between health status and type of morbidity (Szabason 1975) or between health status and risk factors (Aillaud 1976).

In this field CREDOC's work (Rosch 1976) on the construction of a multidimensioned indicator is in many ways original. The purpose is to improve traditional classifications (for instance ICD) by including into the taxonomy different dimensions (symptoms, syndromes, kind of lesion, aetiology) in order to relate each level of health status to a specific network of causes and not only to a main diagnosis.

Regarding the severity of morbid states, the CREDOC indicators (Mizrahi and Rosch 1973), classify into five large categories the forty combinations made from two dimensions of the health state: vital risk and invalidity. However there is a significant statistical link between the two chosen elementary indexes (see Appendix).

The method of attributing scores, moreover, illustrates the lack of consensus research. For the CREDOC authors the fact that only a single physician gives the scores 'makes sure the coherence of judgment'.

As regards scoring, Suchet (Szabason 1975) adopts a similar attitude. Essentially preoccupied with screening a few pathologies, Suchet ends up by constructing a synthetic scale along which individuals can be located whatever disease afflicts them. For each of the 21 selected pathologies there is a number, variable but always small, of quantitative or qualitative biological examinations. Suchet claims that the thresholds are smaller than those generally used, arguing that the purpose of his indicator is to screen and prevent illness, without explaining how he obtains the figures.

In another French study by the DORIA center (Aillaud 1976) the scoring problem consists in defining the degree of positivity of each test (eight for a pathological index, ten for ageing index and six for a social factors index). The authors attribute one to a negative test, two to an insignificant test, three to moderate and four to acute manifestation. The only given explanation is that 'this is of course a conventional weighting but it is useful since it allows comparisons'. Concerning this way of scoring Brun (1975) concludes: 'it is an evaluation in which the intuition of the physician will preponderate'.

De La Roche, in discussing Suchet's indicator, uses almost the same formulation:

> The combination is established in a very empirical way. It squares with a calculated appreciation that any clinician during his every day practice follows his clinical 'bon sens' about the risk incurred by an individual. . . (De La Roche 1979)

No explanation is given to justify the variation in the weights used to measure health status over the five years of Szabason's study: a doubtful reaction is scored one in 1973 but ten in 1978, a pathological reaction is scored four in 1973 but 15 in 1978 and a severely pathological reaction is scored nine in 1973 but 20 in 1979.

On the problem of scaling an elementary index the CREDOC researchers hold that:

> In order to present the results in a 'usable' way we must formulate some hypothesis about the distance between different levels of risk or invalidity. Because of the lack of information we have adopted the simple hypothesis: the distances between the different levels are identical. This does not imply that one can evaluate the difference of invalidity between level a and level b or between c and d; only that the differences are equal. This hypothesis is obviously not entirely tenable – especially in vital risk – where it is probable that the distance between the levels rises with the risk; but one has no basis for saying whether this growth is exponential or algebraic . . . The more simple hypothesis was, in any event, eventually adopted (Mizrahi and Rosch 1973).

A similar attitude is shown towards the aggregation procedure followed to obtain a single indicator. For each component of the DORIA indicator, the final score is obtained by a simple addition of the different scores given by 'the physician's intuition'. The overall indicator is calculated for the whole population by adding the three scores obtained, individually for each index and weighting them as follows: three for pathological, two for ageing and one for social factors.

There is no available evidence presented as to why the values were chosen or the method used to choose them. The authors write: 'In order to characterize an index of the level of health status for different social categories . . . it is necessary to use an approximation. In the present state of our knowledge this approximation can only be arbitrary'. Stephanopoli de Commene, the index inventor, explains: 'If the social test has a weak coefficient it is because social status intervenes indirectly, but decidedly, on other tests'.

In the case of the CREDOC and Suchet indicators a simpler procedure was adopted: the vector of weights is equal to one. So when one compares French studies to the sophistication of most Anglo-Saxon researches (see for instance chapter 3) a larger problem appears: the refusal to use mathematics, which is the general rule of the French work in this territory. It is worth speculating why this should be.

One reason may be a 'cultural distrust' of formal rigour by physicians, who form the majority of contributors. One epidemiologist, Dr Deyme, attributes this mistrust to the Latin culture which is (he believes) historically less inclined to formalization (see also Cayolla da Motta 1979). We thus have physician domination in this new field, coupled with innumeracy.

Another explanation is specific to France. The social status of research in public health — as distinct from health administration — and especially the balkanized structure of the French health system explains why the authors do not generally need to justify the utility of their studies in other areas than the one in and for which they have been carried out. A reason given by two French physicians as to why they did not trouble to test the validity of their indicator is that 'it concerns patients going to visit a physician and they would not have understood why the examination had to be done again by another physician' (Menrad and Colvez 1978). As the reproducibility of results is not a central preoccupation the emphasis is put on results rather than method.

Some general lessons can be drawn from this analysis of French studies. We know that the institutional and sociological background in which researches are carried is very dependent not only on the nature of the topic itself but also on the way the problem, here the multidimensionality of health, is treated. But when methodology and ethics are closely related in a national culture context, this distinctiveness becomes an obstacle to the diffusion of research to other countries. Sophistication, which is consciously avoided by some researchers because often it is nothing but a pseudo-scientific dressing up of subjective values, may in some cases be necessary to make exchanges between researchers easier. On the other hand the use of mathematical or statistical tools must not be an objective *per se*.

In so far as health indicators are to be used for specific purposes, several methodologies must be adapted – in this area there is no 'one best way'.

Some recent Anglo-Saxon studies indicate a growing scepticism toward quantitative techniques (see for instance Doherty and Hicks 1978) which suggests that the attitude adopted by the researchers quoted here may reflect a tendency that might in the near future become more widespread.

Confidence in the subjectivity of a physician's judgment leads to a secondary but not negligible advantage: the low cost of studies. Perhaps choice has actually been guided by such financial considerations. This point is of course made in the French context but recent events lead me to suppose that here too is a matter for international concern!

APPENDIX
INTERDEPENDENCY OF INDEXES: CREDOC INDICATOR (MIZRAHI AND ROSCH 1975)

The two components, vital risk and invalidity, are presented as ordinal scales having respectively five and eight items (Figure 4.1). There are 40 (5 x 8) potential combinations. The sample to which the indicator was applied had the characteristic of being concentrated around the diagonal of the two-way matrix.

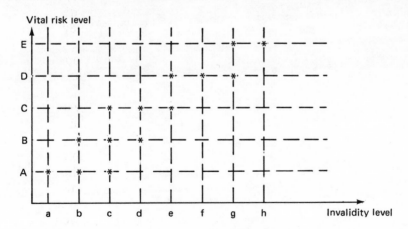

FIG 4.1 *Credoc indicator*

Thus 80 per cent of the population are located on the 14 points, indicated with a cross, representing only 35 per cent of the combinations. The interdependency of the factors thus revealed allows the revelation of a third dimension which is 'anonymous' and one does not know whether it comes more from the subjectivity of the measure than from the characteristics of the sample.

5

Uses and Users of Information in Health Care

J W WEEHUIZEN and H L KLAASSEN

INTRODUCTION

The main question discussed in this paper relates to the relationship of particular types of information to particular users of information: 'who uses what in which activity?'. To answer this question it is necessary to note:

(1) the participants in health care (they are the users of information);
(2) the range of activities of these participants;
(3) the various types of information (for example: a physician needs individualized data in contrast with a health care planning agency which needs a more *aggregated* type of data).

In the paper we give some background on these issues. We start with the participants in health care: the *users* of the information. The next section concentrates on the activities or uses for which the information is assembled, followed by a paragraph containing a classification of information and three basic ways of information-gathering. The closing section of the paper is an attempt to connect the information with activities and participants.

PARTICIPANTS IN HEALTH CARE/USERS OF INFORMATION

Many individuals, institutions, government agencies, and so on, are participating in some form of health care (either as 'consumer' or as 'provider'). These participants in health care are the users of information about health, health status and related fields of interest.

In this paper we are interested only in governmental, institutions and individuals that are related directly to the functioning of the health care system itself (thus including patients, doctors, social security agencies and so on). We exclude for example a Central Bureau of Statistics, being only an intermediate in gathering information, and therefore only indirectly related to the health care system.

The user of information decides on the character of the data he needs for a specific use. As indicated, a broad spectrum of users exists that can be roughly split into a 'demand' side (consumers of health care) and a 'supply' side (providers of health care and related services). On the 'demand' side we will distinguish the 'community as consumers', that is patients and/or groups of patients; parts of the population (for example regional, occupational groups, age, sex); and the population as a whole. On the 'supply-side' generally a distinction can be made between medical practice: persons and institutions that actually cure or prevent illness; and those that are making health care possible by making resources available. In this regard the main participants on the 'supply' side are on the one hand health service providers and the community as provider and, on the other, health-service planners and managers, researchers, teachers, the judiciary, the legislature, and international organisations. One may think that research also can be very close to medical practice (for example in university hospitals). Figure 5.1 presents an overview of these various participants.

Demand

The community is a consumer of health care services in two different ways. In the first place individuals as patients are subject to the curative activities of health service providers. Individual patients need information to make their own best judgements about the range of clinical resources, for example physicians, dentists, hospitals. The necessary data for these choices will probably be of a disaggregated character, as they have to be relevant to the individuals' needs. The type of data, for example, may range from the distance to the doctor's office to the quality of local hospital treatment. Secondly people are subject to preventive activities or 'positive' health care. These activities aim to change the lifestyle of people in such a way as to improve their health (positive health care) or to protect them from diseases (prevention). The information needed in preventive activities is usually aggregated: individuals are not personally directed by the information (for example figures of the prevalence of cancer probably caused by smoking).

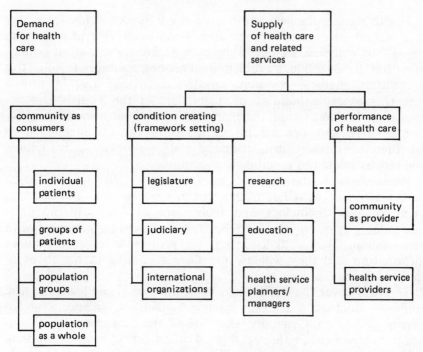

FIG 5.1 *Participants in health care*

Supply

On the supply side of health services are included health service providers like GPs, specialists, dentists, chemists, nurses. These providers actually do the 'curing' and in part are engaged in prevention and positive health care. They need data in determining the best care for specific patients. These data will essentially be of an individualised character. Besides this they also need a theoretical and empirical framework in which a diagnosis can be made.

A second, mostly non-professional, but growing, category of providers is the community itself. Traditionally the family acted as the provider of primary health care. Later this type of health care has been replaced by professional institutions. Recently we have seen a resurgence of roles for the family, neighbourhood and so-called self-help groups. They need both individualized data referring to their own experience and more aggregated data (for example about prevention).

Health service planners and managers are located at local, regional and central government levels. They need to determine where the pay-off to marginal scarce resources is highest. The central government has, for example, a problem in allocating resources to collective prevention, medical research, curative activities, and infrastructure (for example building of hospitals). At the local level other allocation problems arise, for example the total number and distribution of physicians, dentists, physiotherapists. The data planners need are therefore usually institutionally and/or geographically defined and mostly related to specific client-groups.

Researchers in the field of medical and health-related research have a range of activities running from the invention and development of new medicines and techniques of diagnosis and care, determining causes of disease to building models of the national health care system. They actually invent the prototypes of each kind of information and they will use measures according to the focus of their research.

Teachers cover the whole field of health care. They teach medical students, doctors, specialists, chemists, planners, engineers, statisticians, and so on. Generally, they use *all* the data in the health and health-related fields, either aggregated or individual, local or national.

The two categories of the judiciary and the legislature create the basic legislative framework for health care. In general the legislature seeks to frame a legal and constitutional context in which costly but ineffective procedures are not made available. The legislature needs measures enabling it to assess the likely consequences of general rules, terms of access to health services, and so on, for decision-making. The measures themselves are likely often to be specific as regards, say, client groups, but not specific as regards individual persons.

The judiciary has among other things the task of establishing the causes of disabling conditions, in cases where there is, say, negligence by one party that harms the health of another. The judiciary generally needs measures applicable in individual cases brought for adjudication that enable individual decisions to be made regarding, for example fault, fair compensation, injunctions and the like.

The last category is international organizations (for example, WHO). They need information to establish general guidelines of good practice and to give advice to countries, to make international comparisons of different countries' experiences that may be useful to policymaking institutions within member states. International organizations typically need highly aggregated measures relating to health and the health care systems. A special characteristic of these measures is that they have to be standardized to make international comparison possible.

CLASSIFICATION OF ACTIVITIES

The ultimate goal of the activities of these various participants (users of information) is the improvement of health. Activities are therefore excluded that are directly related to profit-making or the survival of firms. However many activities are only indirectly related to the actual practice of curing, (defined as a progress from disability to diagnosis to treatment to recovery or handicap), prevention and positive health care. One could think, for example, of activities directed to the better functioning of the internal organization of the health care system as a whole.

We concentrate here on five activities that mainly have an intermediate function in health care. These activities are allocation (including evaluation), budgeting, compensation, incentives and research. These activities are not of the same level of abstraction. Another classification of activities could have been in terms of the direct output of user categories: for example laws and regulations as an output of legislation; numbers of doctors and nurses as an output of education; medicines, technical devices, finance systems and so on as an output of research. We prefer the former classification because in general these activities are performed by all the participants, although with a different emphasis. We shall return to this later in the paper. No direct connection between the activities (uses) and the participants (users) will be made explicit at this stage. Later an attempt is made to relate users of information to its uses.

Allocation

This is concerned with the allocation of scarce resources to and within health services and the health affecting environment and hence with setting priorities among sectors. The latter implies that allocation includes political values and objectives across a broad spectrum of concerns, even extending beyond the health services as normally conceived.

Before allocation can take place a research process is needed to identify objectives and/or problems and generate and select alternative ways/measures to meet and/or solve them. This process is commonly known as *evaluation*. Evaluation is effectively used by all participants and they are all in one way or another allocators, although the use of the term allocation in medical practice is rather unusual. Two components play a major role in evaluation and allocation: effectiveness and efficiency. Effectiveness is related to an optimal or satisfying distribution of resources, whereby certain goals are sufficiently attained. Efficiency can be described as the ratio of the effective or useful output to the total input in a system.

Capital budgeting

Capital budgeting is particularly concerned with the allocation of scarce resources over time in decisions which involve *current* outlays in return for expectations of *future* benefits. Budgeting in health services and other sectors that effect health is not different from budgeting in other sectors of the economy. Budgeting takes place in all institutions including government. It also occurs in lower tier decision making: for example in primary health care.

Compensation

In one sense compensation refers to payments by for example insurance companies for medical treatment. On the other hand it refers also to making amends for injury, fault etc. In most cases compensation is defined in financial terms.

Incentives

Incentives relate to the possibility of stimulating, coordinating and directing organizations, health service personnel, patients and individuals in the community. Incentives therefore relate to behavioural models of human action in health affecting activities in (and beyond) the health services sector.

Research

We consider research as a typical intermediate activity in health care. Three types of research can be distinguished: medical research, epidemiological research and health services research. Especially of relevance for this paper is the second type. Epidemiology theorises about disability and its causes (individual or due to the environment).

CLASSIFICATION OF INFORMATION/DISAGGREGATIONS

The purpose of this section is to show a possible classification of information that may be useful in health services and derive from it a set of basic information gathering procedures. As has been seen above, users need information of various kinds and at various levels of aggregation. While analysing this information the following categories emerge.

The first category focuses on the *aggregation-disaggregation* issue. Generally stated there are several levels of aggregation in information. The kind of information that is split up in its basic elements is called disaggregated information. Combining these basic elements is called aggregation. A health status indicator is a typical example of aggregated information. Every aggregation procedure causes a loss of information.

The second category relates to the question of whether the information has to describe a phenomenon as a state (isolated from other phenomena) or the relation between two or more phenomena. OECD mentioned in relation with this category three basic disaggregations of main *social* indicators (OECD 1976, Johnston 1977), those by:

(a) ascribed characteristics (for example age, sex);
(b) well-being characteristics, that is to say correlates with other social indicators (for example income, employment status);
(c) contextual variables (for example causes of death, illness and accidents).

The third category relates to the question whether the information is *static* or *dynamic*. By static is meant the situation at a fixed moment of time, and by dynamic the situation during a period of time.

The foregoing categories can be put together as in Figure 5.2, which shows the possible types of information in relation to one another.

At *A* we see static information about the state of a variable on a low aggregation level, that is the description of the state of a small part of a phenomenon at a particular point in time, for example, a patient's blood pressure at a certain moment in time.

In an analogous way we can identify other points of the scheme. It is not continuous in all dimensions, only in level of aggregation and not, for example, in the distinction between static and dynamic.

Gathering information of the above mentioned types causes

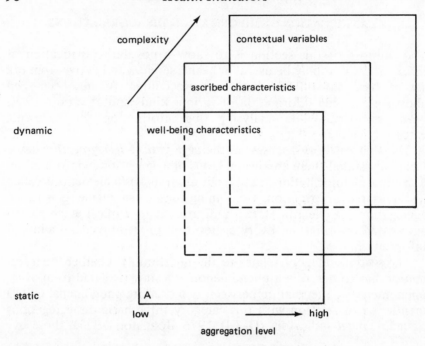

FIG 5.2 *Types of information*

specific problems (for each combination of types of information). On the other hand each type of information has its specific function (use or purpose) in the health care system.

Three basic ways of gathering information may be mentioned. They cover as far as we can see all types of information. These basic ways are as follows:

1. *Observation*, which can be done incidentally, periodically or continuously. Incidental observation produces the state of affairs (the value of a variable). Gathering this information is generally subject to measurement problems, that is a variable needs an operational definition (and an instrument suitable for the measurement). Periodic and continuous observation are commonly known as 'monitoring'.

2. *Prognosis/forecasting*; every action or decision is directed to the change (improvement) of a situation in the future. For that reason information about the future is necessary. Prognosis and forecasting are able to produce this information by, for example, extrapolation of observed trends. The various ways in which

prognosis and forecasting are done in practice are beyond the scope of this paper.

3. *Theorizing*; the third basic way of gathering information we call theorizing or modelling. The kind of theorizing we mean here acts as an input to activities. With respect to health, the theory or models should specify the relationships between health (as measured by several types of indicators) and the variables affecting health in a positive or negative way. Theorizing in this sense shows that researchers also act as an user category.

These techniques for gathering information are basic to the participants in several activities. In the next section we will try to relate information needs of participants to their activities.

PARTICIPANTS-ACTIVITIES-INFORMATION

Hitherto we have identified participants in the health care system, classified their (intermediate) activities, and noted three categories of information. A synthesis of all these components is not possible in this paper because of the numerous combination of participants and activities and even more because of the complexity of the activities and the information needed.

Nevertheless in this section an attempt is made to illustrate in a schematic form the relationship between (some) health service providers, their activities and information needs. In figure 5.3 the various categories of information from the previous section are numbered.

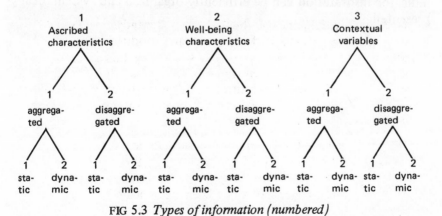

FIG 5.3 *Types of information (numbered)*

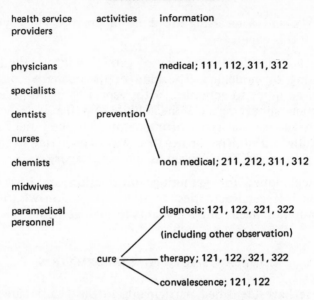

FIG 5.4 *Participants, activities and information*

Figure 5.4 shows the listing of health service providers, their activities and the type of information needed for these activities.

From the consideration of participants, their activities and the information they need it is possible to draw up a complete list of appropriate health indicators. The next step is to categorize these indicators. This will lead to a listing of the same indicators used in the various (different) activities. In such a way, collecting health indicator information can be efficiently organized and systematically presented.

6

What Kind of Health Measure for What Kind of Purpose?

MOGENS NORD-LARSEN

INTRODUCTION

The aim of this paper is to explore the relationship between the various possible purposes for which health status measures may be used and the kind of measure that is needed. This relationship is of particular importance to international organizations like OECD and WHO and, indeed, to all who consider investing substantial sums of money in information systems. Europe stands on the brink of several initiatives of this sort and the present moment is therefore particularly appropriate for these issues to be considered systematically.

The paper starts by discussing the underlying need for measures of health status. After that the connections between definitions of health and methods of measuring health status are discussed. Finally the choice of methods is discussed and some recommendations made.

THE NEED TO MEASURE HEALTH STATUS

Many needs for health status measurement have been pointed out in literature. It seems that eight such needs are generally recognized:

(1) evaluation;
(2) monitoring;
(3) prognosis/forecasting;
(4) allocation;
(5) compensation;
(6) incentives;
(7) budgeting;
(8) theorizing.

Whatever the specific need is, one thing all uses have in common is a need for a useful description of health status in the population studied. By 'description' is meant a general description of the health status of an individual or of a population rather than a description based solely upon the existence or absence of a small range of diagnoses, or a restrictive list of disabilities.

A description may be longitudinal: a time profile in different population groups and in different geographical areas. Some of the eight needs mentioned are met by such time profiles: for example monitoring, forecasting, compensation and perhaps theorising. For needs such as evaluation, allocation and budgeting, descriptions should be related to some kind of evaluation. This raises further problems, dealt with below.

DEFINITION OF HEALTH

Prior to the construction or choice of a method of health status measurement, it is crucial to make clear the concept of health status, so that what is actually measured accords with what has been conceptually defined. The concept has also to be acceptable to researchers, legislators, administrators using the results.

From the literature dealing with measurement of health status it is evident that health is still often defined as 'freedom from disease'. Most of the newer methods for measuring health status, however, are informed by a more sociomedical definition like the WHO definition or Parsons' (1972) definition of health.

As an example of a method very clearly related to the WHO definition of health should be mentioned the measure used in the Alameada County Study (Belloc *et al.* 1973, Breslow 1972). This is an ordinal scale with categories ranging from clear diagnoses through minor complaints to no problems related to illness at all.

The Sickness Impact Profile (SIP) method of measurement (Bergner *et al.* 1976 a and b, Gilson *et al.* 1975, Pollard *et al.* 1976) could be seen as related to Parsons' definition, although his definition is not mentioned at all in the SIP literature. The SIP does not deal at all with the measure or absence of illness but only with 'the extent to which people are able to perform the roles and tasks for which they have been socialized'.

Often there will be no clear indication of the definition underlying a specific method of measurement. It is nonetheless necessary that the potential user of a method analyses the health definition used to ensure the validity of the method in its context.

Even when the definition of health has been chosen for its specific context, problems concerning operationalizing it remain. The problems are especially hard when it is wished to make longitudinal or cross-cultural studies of health status. It is well known that definitions of health and their application have validity only over a short period of time and in specific cultures. Many examples indicate this.

If diagnosis is a part of a health definition, better facilities for making diagnoses mean lower reliability in longitudinal studies. Better treatment facilities cause changes in the conception of illness, for example, in relation to arthritis, which fifty years ago was considered as a normal problem of elderly people but now is regarded as and consequently treated as illness.

If health status is defined by functional capacity or the degree of disability, it is evident that a given illness or handicap causes different problems in Western European society and the Third World. When constructing or choosing methods of measuring health status it is therefore necessary to be aware of to the extent to which it will be used cross-culturally or over periods of time. The more varied the conditions to which the measure is going to be applied, the more universal and the less specific the measure will have to be. Some of these problems have been discussed by Lerner (1973), for example.

METHODS OF DESCRIPTION OF HEALTH STATUS

According to the literature three general types of methods of measurement exist:

(a) descriptions based on diagnostic classification or symptoms of illness;
(b) descriptions based on global subjective values of health status;
(c) descriptions based on functional status or of disability.

These descriptions may apply either at a given time, or over time, or cross-culturally.

Diagnostic and symptomatic classification

The best known of the many existing diagnostic classifications is the International Classification of Diseases (ICD), which is built up from a system of very specific diagnoses. This classification is particularly suitable when facilities are highly developed in, for example, hospitals. If, however, one wants a description of groups of non-institutionalized people, for example, samples of the normal population, one has usually to rely on self-reported data. In this case the ICD classification and other similar classifications lose their usefulness. In Sweden and Denmark — and probably in most other European countries — classifications of diagnoses and symptoms of patients presenting in general practice have been constructed or are under construction. In some of these classifications diagnoses or symptoms can be categorised at more than one level of detailed specificity and the possibility exists of including social problems, difficulties in family relations, and so on. Some of the classifications are constructed in a way that allows self-reported diagnoses and symptoms to be categorized without difficulty. When making descriptions of the health status of large populations, classifications must not be too over-refined so that they become impossible. Thus, if the researcher wants a classification of diagnoses or symptoms incorporated into a description of health status, the best choice seems to be to seek classifications into which self-reported, unspecified and unverified diagnoses can be fitted.

At the same time it is necessary to bear in mind the limitations of self-reported diagnoses. In Sweden it has been shown that people who estimate their health status as generally fine under-report their visits to physicians while, on the contrary, people with a general feeling of illness overestimate visits. Experience in Denmark — which has a well-established primary health care system — shows relatively little variation between diagnoses obtained in health interviews and physicians' knowledge of their patients. Anyway it would be dangerous to overestimate the reliability of self-reported data on health matters.

Finally, we have to call in question the use of diagnosis itself as a description of health status in a population. Diagnoses are obviously part of the picture of health status, but if one counts only diagnoses, one is restricting oneself to a kind of dichotomy: 'sick' or 'not sick'. We cannot tell whether a man with two diagnoses is better off than a man with three. Diagnoses give no knowledge of severity, loss of functional ability, and so on. Diagnosis itself is not an adequate description of health status.

Global subjective valuation of health status

Under this heading are questions and responses like:

How do you estimate your health in general?
Excellent/good/poor/very bad.

This kind of measure has shown a fairly good correlation with a vector of other factors that are normally accepted as parts of a description of state of health (Maddox 1964). However, this method of measurement cannot be used in relation to the needs listed at the beginning of this paper because it is uncertain what precisely is being measured. On the other hand this kind of global measure could be of some value as an easy valuation of health status in social research with no special socio-medical approach.

Measures of function or disability

As stated earlier a set of new measures of disability has been constructed during the last ten years, probably as a consequence of the recognized weakness of diagnoses or symptoms as measures of health status and the acceptance of more sociomedical definitions of health. The first disability indices − like the original Katz's Activities of Daily Living (ADL) index (Katz *et al.* 1963, 1976) − seem to have been constructed for evaluating treatment in relation to specific diagnoses or patient groups and they therefore concentrated on disabilities specific for those groups. As the sociomedical definition of health has become more widely accepted, disability measures including more dimensions of the daily living have been constructed and accepted as useful descriptions of health status. If measures have to be used for description of health status of people both with and without illness, they have to discriminate in both the negative and the positive part of the health continuum. As a result, measures of disability can to a large extent be seen as measures of quality of life.

Most of the disability measures are on ordinal scales. This is true for example of Katz's ADL index, of the measure in the Health Insurance Study (HIS) (Steward *et al.* 1978), and in the Alameada County Study (Belloc *et al.* 1973). Fewer measures have been cardinal: the best known example is the Sickness Impact Profile (Bergner *et al.* 1976). The cardinal scale naturally has the greatest scope in analysis; however, questions can and will be raised concerning the validity of the weights employed. This problem also arises when using cardinal measures in cross-cultural or longitudinal studies when the weights applicable in one place or time may be inapplicable in another. Whether for this or other reasons, ordinal scales tend to be more generally accepted (although there also might be problems using them cross-culturally or over time).

One of the greatest problems in the use of measures of disability is the association between disability and factors in the surrounding environment. Whether an individual is able to work, to travel or to live in his own home depends not only on his own disability but also on other factors in the society in which he lives. If researchers are not aware of this, they might be measuring the effects of, say, unemployment benefit rather than any job-disabling aspect of an individual's ability to function. For use in longitudinal and cross-cultural studies it is necessary to seek measures that are as far as possible independent of such social factors.

What should health status describe?

If one accepts a sociomedical definition of health, measures of disability offer the best approach to describing health status. The reason for this is obviously that disability measures, in contrast with diagnostic or symptomatic data, give information about how health status affects the quality of life in a variety of ways. Moreover from a practical point of view, disability measures are most readily applied to populations.

On the other hand the researcher will often be in need of finding a link between diagnosis and disability. If, as an example, one is concerned with allocating resources for treatment, the decision maker ought to know how much disability is related to what kind and what number of diagnoses.

It seems generally desirable that in describing health status one should carefully consider the need for *both* a measure of disability *and* of using the diagnostic conditions giving rise to the disability. Where, in specific cases, the emphasis should lie will depend, of course, on the circumstances of the case: there is no general rule that defines as to where weight should be placed.

PROBLEMS SPECIALLY RELATED TO USE OF HEALTH STATUS MEASURES IN EVALUATION

As mentioned above the use of health status measures in evaluation raises some specific problems. For the subsequent discussion it would be practical to split up the concept of evaluation in two parts that are not quite mutually exclusive but are nonetheless useful:

(1) evaluation of specific health services at the micro level, related to specified diagnoses or other health problems;
(2) evaluation of health services in general, of health policies or of health services in relation to nonspecific illness.

Evaluation of health services in relation to specified diagnoses

We assume that the context is that of a study in which the objective is:

(1) evaluation of a well-defined treatment or other well-defined service;
(2) in relation to one or a few well-defined diagnoses;
(3) in a well-defined population;
(4) normally of small size;
(5) with the possibility of a control group.

Evaluation of treatment of acute conditions will normally involve only the use of clinical or paraclinical data, and shall not be discussed here.

In evaluating treatment of chronic diseases the researcher is in need of both clinical data and a measure of disability. In most cases wide measures like SIP or HIS will not be the best choice. They will often be insufficiently discriminating in relation to the problems caused by the illness or the effects of the treatment that is to be evaluated. The researcher then has to establish or to seek measures relevant to the specific disability caused by the specific illness.

Apart from the original ADL index, this kind of specific disability measures is not much discussed in the literature. On the other hand, a great potential for making such measures must exist because of the great experience of physicians, nurses and other personnel working with people having well-defined diagnoses, the treatment of which is going to be evaluated. As an example, sexual functioning and changes in it might be a hitherto mostly unused part of a measure of disability in relation to cardiovascular diseases.

Evaluation of general health services in relation to non-specific illness

Examples of this type of evaluation could be:

(1) evaluation of general environmental policies to promote health (for example clean air, industrial safety legislation);
(2) evaluation of alternative financing systems in terms of health outcomes;
(3) evaluation of non-diagnostic categories (for example home-helps).

The measures of health status to be used in this kind of evaluation do not differ much from the measures to be used in the pure description of health status. Since we do not deal with specified diagnosis we will be in need of broad-ranging measures.

Since there will often be no possibility of control-groups, the measures have to be used in 'before and after situations', or in some kind of multivariate analysis.

At the practical level it is appropriate to be sceptical about the evaluation of general health services or general health policy. The fact that health status is related to a lot of factors besides health services, and the fact that health services are generally extensively provided in the European countries means that it will be very difficult to use existing measures to detect any effects of alterations in health services or in health policy. At its worst it could mean that health service provision would be cut because existing measures are not sensitive enough to changes in levels of provision.

RECOMMENDATIONS

The current state of the art has not yet reached a point where it is possible to point to measures appropriate for measuring health status in every context. Much work remains to be done, particularly to evaluate expert valuations of health status so as to avoid the extensive dependence on self-reported data, the reliability of which should be questioned.

Given the current state of the art the following six general precepts are offered in the hope that they may help one to choose an appropriate procedure in any specific case.

(1) Specify the purpose of the measurement. Are you just going to make some kind of a description of health status as background for monitoring or forecasting, and so on or is the measure to be used in evaluation and if so, of what kind?
(2) Specify the population whose health status you are going to

study. If you are talking about a sample of the normal population, you will need disability measures that discriminate also in relation to the positive part of the health continuum. If you are talking of populations with specified diagnoses, you will need measures discriminating in relation to problems caused by specific diseases.

(3) Specify how many resources you will be able to spend in terms of money, size of questionnaire, time for preparing your own method of measurement.

(4) You will normally need both a disability measure and a classification of diagnoses or symptoms. How wide the disability measure has to be depends on the population studied (as mentioned under (2)). If you are going to evaluate some specified treatment, you need a disability measure (besides the clinical and paraclinical data) that in particular takes into consideration the disability caused by the illness whose treatment you want to evaluate.

(5) If you need a disability measure, you must seek for one of those very few that has been evaluated seriously and has been used frequently. Among measures giving a wide and positively-orientated description, the SIP is especially worthy of evaluation. Among other methods of measurement that have been frequently used (but perhaps more orientated towards sick people and less discriminating) are the HIS and the method of measuring in the Alameada County Study. Measures concentrating on disability caused by specific illness, usable in evaluation of treatment, are seldom quoted in the literature. As pointed out earlier, there might exist a large number of such disability measures that could be standardized through use.

(6) Whatever you do — be careful!

7

The Need for Health Indicators

AINA UHDE

INTRODUCTION

Before exploring some details of health indicator construction the
use to which such indicators may be put is discussed. The aim of
health indicators is to measure health status, and they may apply to
a heterogenous population group, a group of people with a specific
disease or a single person. In the following the discussion is restricted
to measures summarizing health status at an aggregate level. The
discussion will be restricted to viewing health indicators as a tool of
improving public decision-making. Measuring health status for its
own sake seems of little importance.

Interest in health indicators has developed out of recent attempts
to build a system of social accounts describing relationships between
resources provided for the social sector and their effects. Advocates
of a social accounts system regard it as a necessary supplement to the
familiar system of national accounts, for although resources allocated
to the social sector are included in the national accounts system, any
outcome of the activity in this sector is not accounted for. It is
argued that just as economists have constructed the concept of GNP
expressing the total value of economic activity during a year, one
should construct concepts valuing the activity devoted to reducing
health and other social problems. A single measure for health status
in the population is therefore sought. We shall discuss below the
problems involved in obtaining such a gross measure in the absence
of a set of prices allowing aggregation of the different components.

The natural economic interpretation of how such a measure of
health status would be used would be in an optimizing framework
where overall policy was postulated to have as its objective the
maximization of social welfare. Social welfare would be seen as
dependent not only on the traditional economic measures of well-

being such as per capita consumption, but also on other measures such as health status. Such a model would include both the determinants of health status (for example the way in which it was affected by production and consumption patterns in the economy), and how health status itself had feedback effects on the economy (for example as a determinant of aggregate labour supply).

In such a (somewhat ambitious) analysis the health status measure would enter both the objective function and the two types of structural relationships mentioned. In practice, a single indicator of health may be both impossible to obtain and, anyway, be too highly aggregated: separate indicators for mortality and morbidity will be needed. One reason for this is that consumption enters the welfare function on a per capita basis. The model must therefore distinguish between changes in population size and changes in morbidity. Another is that the labour supply function may need to treat the effects of changes in mortality and morbidity separately.

In the next section the need for health indicators is discussed in a more partial and less ambitious context. However, it may be instructive to see these more practical uses in the light of the 'ideal' optimization procedure that has been briefly outlined above.

THE NEED FOR HEALTH INDICATORS

In practice health indicators may be used (1) to reveal the time trend of health status or the distribution of health status among population groups, (2) to examine factors affecting the health of the population, and (3) to determine resource allocation to health programmes.

Good health is sometimes referred to as a 'merit good' and often specified as a separate argument in the welfare function in models dealing with health care. This indicates that politicians are assumed to have a special concern for the general status of health in the population. If so, it would be most desirable if health status could be expressed by a single indicator. In this way, an unfavourable time trend of health could more quickly be brought to the policy makers' attention than would the presentation of various time trends for disaggregated measures. A general health indicator would also serve international comparisons, although these may be of less importance for policy making on a national level. In addition to a general indicator, indicators revealing differences in health status between social classes and geographical regions would be desirable as a basis for policy making.

Besides a description of the state of health in the population, specific policy actions must also be based on a detailed knowledge of the factors affecting the state of health. Thus, we must try to investigate parts of the structural model briefly sketched above, even if it is not intended to use it in an optimization procedure. Estimation of the causal relationships between on the one hand factors describing the environment, level of education, types of work, sex, amount of health services etc. and, on the other hand, the state of health, requires some aggregate health indicator. Depending upon the level of aggregation a health indicator for the population at large or for a specific subgroup may be needed.

The third type of use for health indicators is in choosing specific policies. A choice among alternative policies to improve the status of health must take account both of their effect upon health and their net cost to society. While the net cost of a specific health policy can be measured in money terms, the change in health status (that is the non-economic effects) attributable to the policy in question must be measured by some kind of health indicator.

The net cost to society of a specific health care programme is defined as consumption forgone due to the programme minus consumption created by the programme. The first of these terms reflects the use of resources in the programme. The second term reflects production created by the increase in available working time. Since both terms are actually time streams, they must be evaluated at their present value by discounting.

In cost-effectiveness analysis, programmes are compared that are assumed to have the same effect upon the health of a specific population group. The problem is to determine which of the alternative programmes can be provided at the lowest net cost to society. For such an analysis a health indicator is needed in order to select programmes with the same effect upon health.

It is quite another question whether the programme having the lowest cost should be provided. To answer this the net cost to society must be weighed against the positive effect on health. This is cost-benefit analysis. However, the effect on health is not simply a higher value of whatever health indicator is used. It is the *difference* between two time profiles of the health indicator — with and without the health programme provided. Policy makers should be asked whether this change in the time stream of health is worth the net social cost involved. They must compare the net cost measured in money terms with the effect on health measured by some health indicator. If politicians had revealed prior evaluations of health measured in money terms, the evaluation of appropriate comparisons could be left to the research worker. Therefore, whether a health indicator *expressed in money terms* is needed depends upon the form in which results are presented to policy makers. If definite recommendations are to be presented as to which health programmes should be provided, the health indicator should be measured in money terms.

It should be stressed that in most cost-benefit analyses, costs and benefits are defined differently from those described above. Usually the cost component includes only the cost of providing the health programme (that is the consumption forgone) while the benefit component includes increased future incomes (that is the consumption created). In addition to this economic benefit, the non-economic benefits are included to a greater or lesser extent, depending upon the difficulties involved in finding adequate measures. However, when presenting the results of the analyses these non-economic benefits are often unintentionally suppressed or completely left out. This may help to account for the negative attitude towards cost-benefit analyses that is to be found among many research workers in the field – even some economists. It seems more in line with the purpose of health care to regard the non-economic health effects as belonging to the benefit side and the net economic effects (consumption forgone minus consumption created) to the cost side (This view is taken in Uhde (1977), and is also suggested in Fanshel and Bush (1970)). In some cases this cost side may of course show up as negative.

Misunderstandings often occur about how the evaluation of health changes forms an important part of any cost-benefit analysis. Some authors, for example, Balinsky and Berger (1975), seem to believe that the evaluation of health changes according to some health indicator is an alternative and more successful procedure for determining resource allocation than by using cost-benefit principles. As emphasized above, the use of health indicators for a concise description of the health effects of a programme should be an integral part of *every* cost-benefit analysis. Cost-benefit analysis is more, not less, comprehensive than the alternative by virtue of the fact that it encompasses *both* the benefit *and* the cost sides.

Before concluding this section it should be mentioned that a correctly specified cost-benefit analysis carried out for a small programme may under certain conditions lead to the same resource allocation as an optimization of the complete model briefly outlined in section 1 (for a mathematical proof, see Uhde (1977)).

SOME PROBLEMS ATTACHED TO HEALTH INDICATORS

The health indicator most used in practice for describing health status at the aggregate level is a summary measure of mortality. It expresses life expectancy at a particular age and for each sex separately. This indicator may be satisfactory for crude comparisons over time or between nations. However, if used alone it is not very satisfactory for evaluating the impact on health of specific health programmes. As a single indicator it is too insensitive since it says nothing about changes in morbidity due to the programmes.

Indicators have therefore been proposed for describing morbidity in the population. Most used is probably the total number of work-loss days or bed-disability days during a given period of time. Clinical disability ratings based on subjective judgements by physicians are less useful for aggregate descriptions. However, when using number of days absent from work as an indicator for comparing morbidity over time or between different groups one must be aware of the danger of measuring instead the impact of income compensation schemes during sickness. This indicator does not describe, moreover the health of that part of the population outside the labour force. Indicators based upon interview data and counting the number of bed-disability days or restricted-activity days may give a more reliable description of health. For all the summary morbidity measures mentioned there is a built-in ethical judgment that society is indifferent between one person being sick for 30 days and 30 persons being sick for one day. This may seem arbitrary but in practice probably difficult to avoid when working with aggregate measures. Alternative weights would also necessarily include subjective judgments.

For many purposes it would of course be convenient to have a combined mortality and morbidity indicator for measuring the status of health. Several indicators have been proposed, of which the best known is that proposed by Sullivan (1971): expected years of life free of disability. The built-in ethical judgments are here even more sweeping and arbitrary than for the morbidity indicators mentioned above. The indicator implies that society is indifferent between one year confined to bed and the loss of one year of life. The indicator further implies that society is indifferent between the loss of one year of life for a young and for an old person, and between the loss of one year of life for 30 persons and the loss of 30 years for one person. These are very serious assumptions and hardly likely to conform to social preferences (defined for example as the preferences held by policy makers).

The subjective judgments underlying combined mortality and morbidity indicators make such indicators valueless for policy purposes. If a combined indicator is wanted, it would be more satisfactory to make this a weighted average (or some other specified functional form) of separate mortality and morbidity indicators, with the weights determined so as to represent social preferences. The morbidity indicator used should preferably also be more elaborate than those mentioned above.

At the present stage of research on health indicators it seems advisable to provide policy makers with rather simple mortality and morbidity indicators together with net cost calculations for specific health programmes. It is then up to policy makers to apply their own weightings in deciding which programmes to offer. Even if the ultimate goal is to measure health in monetary terms, to facilitate comparisons with net costs and provide policy makers with definitive answers the construction of simple indicators may serve as a good starting point. In deciding which indicators would be most valuable to provide one must try to balance two conflicting desiderata: on the one hand the indicators should give policy makers a clearer picture of the health effects than would a set of disaggregated data; on the other, the indicators should not be so aggregated that policy makers lose information which is important for decision taking.

As mentioned earlier, it would be useful to have estimates of the weights applied by policy makers to different health states and groups of population. Thereby, the effect on health from specific health programmes could be measured in money terms and directly compared to the net cost. Several procedures have been proposed for obtaining an evaluation of health in money terms: interviews with policy makers, revealed preferences from actual public decisions, court compensations, wage differentials for work with different health risks, interviews to ascertain people's willingness to pay, and health insurance premiums. Of these alternative procedures the revealed preference approach seems most adequate, since it is the only one that reflects decisions taken by policy makers, that reflects actual behaviour in allocating scarce resources and that is independent of the wealth and income of the people affected.

Although the revealed preference approach should be regarded as theoretically satisfactory, it is in practice very difficult to apply. An objection of principle has also been raised against applying the procedure at the present time: information about the economic and health effects of a programme is usually presented to policy makers unsystematically and, in any case, decision makers frequently seek technical advice interpreting revealed preferences from observed decisions in the past. However, their presentation may make policy makers more aware of past evaluations and enable them explicitly to reconsider them in future decisions.

CONCLUSIONS

At the present time much can be improved in public decisions in the health field by making more information available to policy makers. This will require both more statistical data and more analyses of the economic and health effects of particular programmes. In presenting this information the use of relatively simple health indicators will be most valuable. In the longer term, challenging research lies in investigating social preferences for particular states of health and groups in the population.

8

A Health Statistics Framework: US Data Systems as a Model for European Health Information?

PENNIFER ERICKSON, KLAUS-DIRK HENKE

and ROGER DEAN BRITTAIN

INTRODUCTION

In Europe, health care expenditures are increasing at rates similar to those of the United States. At the same time, resources are becoming increasingly scarce. In view of rising expenditures and shrinking resources, the efficiency of the health care system is being questioned. Thus, policy makers are looking for better health statistics and resource allocation techniques to analyze the effectiveness of the health care sector. As the tightening of resources can be expected to continue, policy makers will need more and better information for decision making. Furthermore, the public's increasing demands for health reinforce policy makers' needs for impartial data.

The development of health data systems in Europe has received low priority in the past. Most data that are available on the delivery of health care are obtained from administrative reporting systems, are not easily disaggregated or are available only for selected sub groups of the population. As a result, these data are of limited value for setting national priorities or for evaluating health programmes. European countries have recently begun to examine the health indicators information systems of the Western world, particularly those of the United States. There is widespread belief that the American system, which is very comprehensive, could serve as a model for some of the European countries.

This paper focuses on health statistics in a policy context. Not only are the functions of health statistics considered but also a framework is proposed according to which health statistics can be grouped. Within this framework, US health statistics are reviewed as to their functional and their organizational purposes. As some information regarding the costs of data collection is included, the paper opens the way for a cost-benefit perspective in regard to having more and better health statistics. The framework can be used by countries to assess the adequacies of their current health statistics data systems and to identify new data sources to meet their policy needs. Thus, the framework with the least cost is particularly important for countries that are considering expanding their data collection activities to include routine health surveys and other types of population-based data.

PURPOSES OF HEALTH INDICATOR INFORMATION SYSTEMS

Functions of Health Statistics

Apart from use in research and teaching, the following objectives of health statistics can be listed: (1) monitoring of health trends; (2) projecting problems and needs in health care; (3) setting priorities and selecting strategies; (4) managing programmes; (5) evaluating programmes and assessing the overall impact of health policy; and (6) educating the public and changing private behaviour. These functions refer to the use of health data in all levels of government as well as in health-related institutions.[1] These functions are not specific to health data; rather, statistics in other areas of concern, such as education, housing, and transportation, have similar uses. However, the framework put forth in this paper is specific to statistics for the health care sector.

Health statistics in a conceptual and policy context. One approach to organizing health statistics is to examine how existing statistics have been used in the past and how they have changed or influenced health policy decisions. On the basis of this information, an information system could be developed according to the uses of its actual and potential clients, for example, voters, researchers, decision makers, planners, and administrators.[2] It would be interesting to compare such consumer-oriented systems with existing systems to observe whether more and better knowledge about the health sector leads, in the course of time, to the collection of different sets of data. In other words, 'how elastic or dynamic is the supply of official health statistics to the changing views and interests of clients?'.

A different approach is based on the premise that the purpose of health statistics information systems is to assess the population's health status. Figure 8.1 identifies some variables that affect the health status of a population. Such a figure can suggest interlinkages but cannot actually state the interactions since the exact relationships are unknown (Auster *et al.* 1972). In addition, but not shown on this figure, the determinants are interlinked with one another. Therefore, figure 8.1 serves as a common-sense approach of analysing the health status of the population and its determinants.

In the climate of shrinking resources, the role of the health care system in improving health status has important policy considerations. If one considers that all of the elements of the health system are aimed at improving the health status of the population, then the question arises 'To what extent does the health care system have a positive effect on the people's health status?'.[3] If medical care should be ineffective for certain population subgroups, for example the elderly, then a second question arises, 'Can a more relevant basis for organizing health indicators be identified that includes, for example, nutrition, environment, housing and working conditions, and life style?'[4]

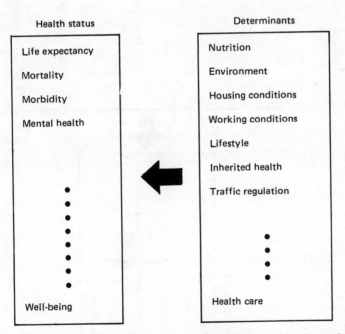

FIG 8.1 *Suggested interlinkages between health status and its determinants*

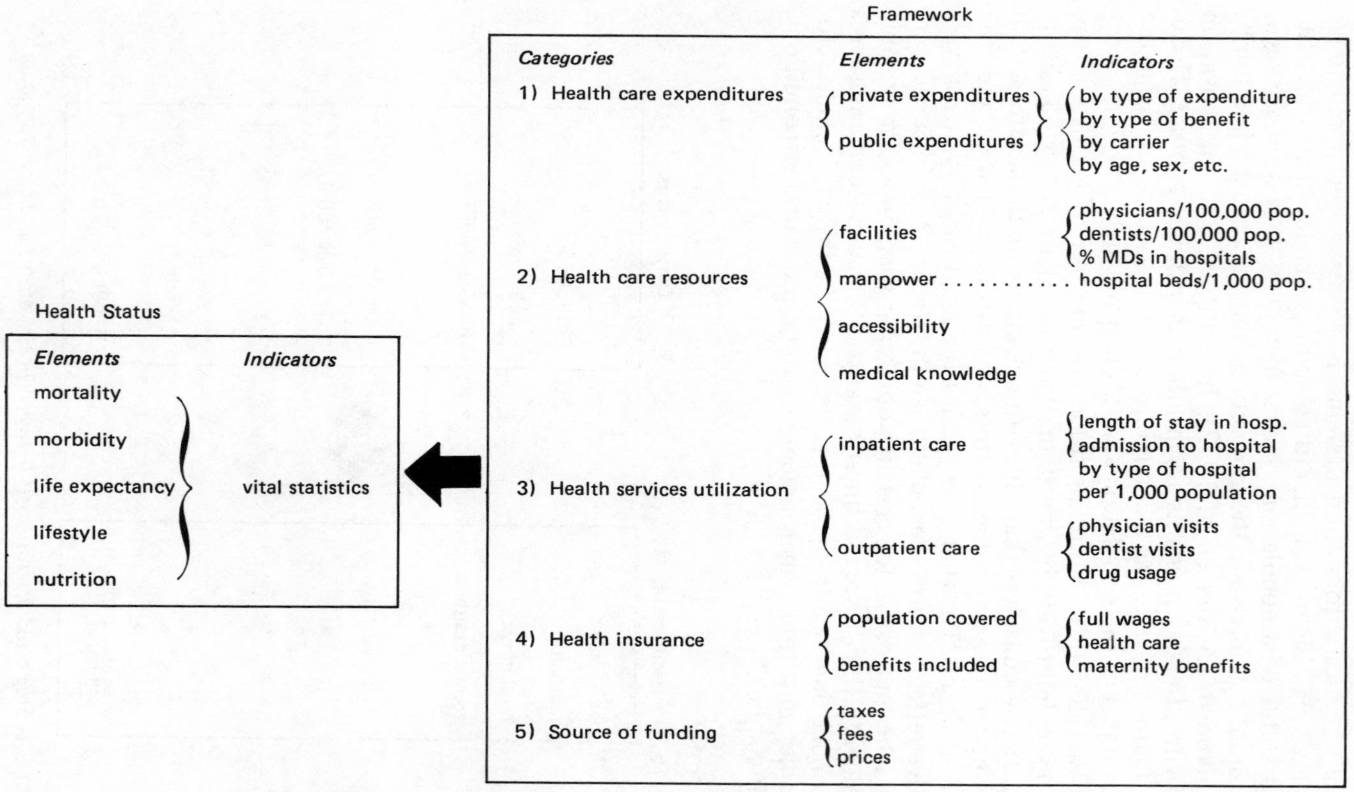

Framework

Categories	Elements	Indicators
1) Health care expenditures	private expenditures public expenditures	by type of expenditure by type of benefit by carrier by age, sex, etc.
2) Health care resources	facilities manpower · · · · · · · · · accessibility medical knowledge	physicians/100,000 pop. dentists/100,000 pop. % MDs in hospitals hospital beds/1,000 pop.
3) Health services utilization	inpatient care outpatient care	length of stay in hosp. admission to hospital by type of hospital per 1,000 population physician visits dentist visits drug usage
4) Health insurance	population covered benefits included	full wages health care maternity benefits
5) Source of funding	taxes fees prices	

Health Status

Elements	Indicators
mortality morbidity life expectancy lifestyle nutrition	vital statistics

FIG 8.2 *Health care delivery system by framework categories showing selected elements and indicators*

A Framework for Health Statistics

Assuming that health care is a major determinant of health status and that its ultimate goal is the improvement of people's health, it is proposed that statistics be organized by subject matter so as to develop further a theory of input-output processes in health care. For this purpose, the production process ('social production function') in health care has been divided into the following five categories: (1) health care expenditures; (2) health care resources; (3) health services utilization; (4) health insurance; and (5) source of funding. This framework includes all levels of analysis in the field of health services research. Within each of the main categories, information on health care system can be further disaggregated into elements.[5] The framework, along with selected elements and indicators of the health care system, is given in figure 8.2.

By further disaggregation, this framework can be extended in a policy context to provide information as to who are the persons, agencies, or carriers that govern the elements in the five categories. For example, in the area of health manpower (an element which falls under category 2), statistical indicators provide information for determining who is making decisions about the levels of education and employment for doctors, nurses, etc. This is just one example of how the framework can provide further information as to the variables that influence the different levels of health care.

Detailed breakdowns by population subgroups are vital for policy purposes, especially since health care policy seems to be moving toward focusing on special population groups, for example, the elderly, children, and the handicapped. At the same time, such summaries, a perhaps unique characteristic of the comprehensive US health statistics system, have the advantage in that they allow both more information and explanation of causal relationships and tests of hypotheses. To better serve people and their needs, disaggregated data are a prerequisite. The following are a sample of topical breakdowns: (1) population groups (elderly, children, handicapped); (2) problem areas (cost containment, quality assessment, access to care); or (3) specific diseases (hypertension, arthritis, rheumatism). For each subgroup, a figure similar to figure 8.2 could be prepared with the elements and indicators being specific to the population. With this information, health administrators and analysts gain further insight into the decision making processes of the participants in the health care sector, for example, the patients, the providers, and the regulators.

Source of information

Elements and indicators	Surveys		Vital statistics	Reporting systems	
	Ongoing	One-time		Reportable disease data registers	Administrative record systems
Mortality					
Life expectancy			●		
Crude mortality rate			●		
Infant mortality			●		
Standardized rate			●		
Morbidity					
Specific diseases (e.g., tuberculosis, heart cancer)	●	●		●	●
Disability (e.g., bed days, limited activity)	●	●			
Disability free life	●	●	●		
Nutrition	●				
Well-being					
Self assessed health status	●	●			

FIG 8.3 *Elements and indicators of health status in the United States Department of Health and Human Services by Source of information*

THE US HEALTH STATISTICS SYSTEM

Sources of information

Health data in the American system are obtained from two primary sources. One source, perhaps that which distinguishes the US system from those in Europe, is the on-going or one-time special-purpose health survey which may be based on a sample or on a total population. Survey information can be obtained from questionnaire, interview, or examination, or from various types of medical records.[6] The other source, one which is commonly used throughout the world, is the continuous or periodic reporting system. Included in this type of health data are: (1) vital statistics, deaths, births, marriages and divorces; (2) reportable diseases such as tuberculosis and measles; and, (3) administrative or regulatory data which are collected primarily for some specific purpose. For example, data from the US Medicare programme files which have been collected for paying medical bills of the beneficiaries provide limited information about health services utilization.

The Framework and the US Data

Health status information collected by these two sources includes measures of the nature and extent of diseases, disability, discomfort, attitudes and knowledge concerning health, and perceived health status as well as need for health care and health services of persons and populations. Figure 8.3 shows elements of health status and health behaviour with some common indicators by source of information. These indicators are available for policy making at the national or federal level.[7] In addition to this information on health status, there is a limited amount of data that describe the end results of the health services provided. Most of these data on health outcomes have been collected from surveys of the general population.

Data on health care expenditures show the costs of health care and the price the population pays to receive medical services. In addition, with rapidly rising expenditures, there is increasing interest in the analysis of costs, prices, charges and payments. These input indicators are furthermore used in comparisons with the health status of a nation to show the overall efficiency of the system. In the US, expenditure data are collected primarily by administrative records but recently national health surveys have been conducted to assess financial aspects of the health care system. These surveys have been implemented to provide inputs into the debates concerning adoption of a national health insurance plan.

Health care resources data that describe health personnel, institutions, agencies, and facilities are obtained primarily from licensure, certification, and other records and periodic inventories. These data are primarily collected by administrative records. Medical and claims records, as well as surveys, provide information about the volume of use and the persons utilizing services. These records also describe health care personnel, facilities, institutions and agencies.

Information on health insurance shows how the population is covered in case of illness and what benefits are included in the health insurance plans. In addition to data from the providers, health insurance information is collected periodically on a probability sample of the general population. Finally, statistics on the source of funding show which population groups bear the burden of health care expenditures. These data are obtained primarily from administrative records.

Disaggregation by Target Population

The levels of disaggregation required for different policy questions vary depending on the nature of the policy to be set, that is, more or less information is required about the subgroups of the target population(s). In general, survey data, whether on-going or special-topic, provide greater levels of disaggregation. From the US National Health Interview Survey, it is possible to obtain information on various disability measures by at least six sociodemographic characteristics: age, race, sex, income, educational status, and geographic location. Similarly, the Master Facility Index provides information on facilities by at least five variables: specialty, number of beds, number of employees, occupancy rate, and number of residents.[8] Since the majority of the administrative data which is collected is used for operating the actual health programme, the amount of data in these systems that is also suitable for national policy making is small. Thus, the specific variables for disaggregation differ depending on the category within the framework, yet the concept of disaggregation is basic to the use of health statistics for decision making.

Organizational Structure

In the US, responsibility and authority for statistical activities are highly decentralized, thus it is difficult to give a clear picture of the activities.[9] Data are collected by various agencies within the Federal government to meet the programmatic needs of the agencies, that is, programme administration, research, and regulation as well as policy-making.[10] While the variety of uses and collection points for the data results in duplication, it also provides a wide range of information about the health care delivery system.

Figure 8.4 shows the health data collection components in the executive branch of the US government which has responsibilities for health data policy, collection or coordination. The largest collector of health data is the Department of Health and Human Services (DHHS). The organizational structure of this department is shown in Figure 8.5; a glossary of acronyms and a brief description of the agencies statistical activities are given in Appendices A and B, respectively.[11] While the majority of the data systems in DHHS collect data for programme management, regulation and research purposes, the National Center for Health Statistics (NCHS) collects general-purpose, population-based health data as mandated in the National Health Survey Act of 1954. As a result of this act, three surveys were established: (1) the National Health Interview Survey which provides information as to the impact of morbidity on the population; (2) the National Health Examination Survey which provides detailed information about physical conditions of the population; and (3) the National Hospital Discharge Survey which collects information on the health care facilities in the nation. Since the passage of the National Health Survey Act, other data systems that collect information about health status, health services utilization, resources and expenditures have been established within NCHS.[12]

Recently it has become apparent that new measures, particularly more sensitive measures of health itself, are needed to monitor the changing impacts that the health care system as well as other determinants have on health status. Specifically, policy makers are looking for measures, such as health indices, which reflect the positive side of health as well as the changing disease and death patterns, such as mortality rates; a health index has been defined as a measure that summarizes data from two or more components and which purports to reflect the health status of an individual or defined group. To promote the development and application of these measures, the Clearing-house on Health Indices was established. Within the last two years an increasing number of research projects which describe the development and/or application of health indexes have appeared in the European literature. Thus, the Clearinghouse is establishing a

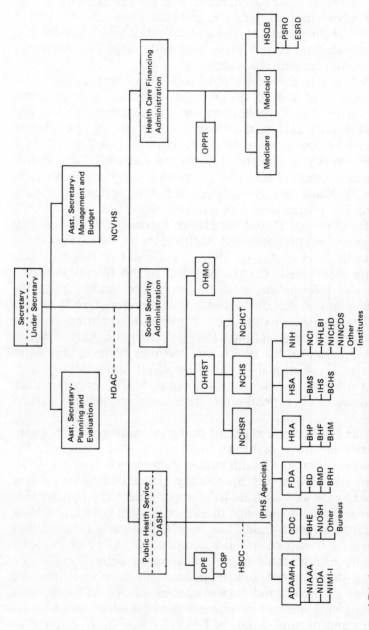

* This diagram depicts only those parts of HHS that have major responsibilities for health data policy, collection, or coordination.
# Full names of components are given in the Glossary of Acronyms
Code: ——— Internal Advisory Committee   xxxxxx External Advisory Committee
Source: Selected topics in Federal Health Statistics, Office of Technology Assessment, Congress of the United States, Washington DC, 1979

FIG 8.4 Federal executive branch components involved in health data activities*

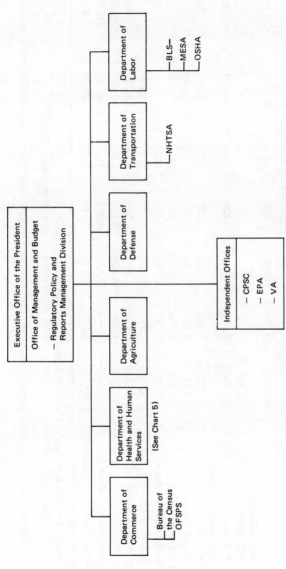

* This diagram depicts only those parts of the executive branch that have major responsibilities for health data policy, collection, or coordination.

Full Names of components are given in the Glossary of Acronyms

Source: Selected Topics in Federal Health Statistics, Office of Technology Assessment, Congress of the United States, Washington, DC, 1979.

FIG 8.5 *Organizational components involved in health data activities**

Agency	Total	Health status	Health resources				Financial	Other
			Total	Facility	Manpower	Utilization		
			(Dollars in thousands)					
Total	119,282	60,028	17,066	11,823	5,243	25,181	13,725	3,282
Office of Assistant Secretary for Planning and Evaluation	2,450							2,450
Public Health Service	95,555	58,498	10,762	5,632	5,130	15,407	10,200	832
Alcohol, Drug Abuse and Mental Health Administration	14,958	7,469	1,585	1,508	77	5,189	85	630
Center for Disease Control	4,225	4,084	94	94		47		
Food and Drug Administration	2,618	1,755	607	329	278	110		146
Health Resources Administration	1,182	19	1,158	128	1,030		5	
Health Services Administration	3,033	288	165	13	152	2,640		
National Institutes of Health	35,223	30,430	827	501	326	3,750	160	
Office of Assistant Secretary for Health	34,316	14,369	6,326	3,059	3,267	3,671	9,950	56
Health Care Financing Administration	12,412		5,128	5,015	113	4,239	3,045	
Office of Human Development Services	8,864	1,674	1,176	1,176		5,535	480	

1 Includes research and evaluation projects which include a large data collection component.
Source: Health Statistics Plan, Fiscal Years 1979–1980, DHEW, Public Health Service, Washington, DC, 1979

FIG 8.6 *Distribution of reported expenditures for heath statistics projects and systems by subject and agency, 1978*

regional information centre in Copenhagen, Denmark. This centre will collect information about health index research throughout Europe, disseminate publications on health indices to persons interested in measuring health status, and provide a library at the Institute of Social Medicine, University of Copenhagen for easy access by European researchers.[13]

Costs of the US System

Due to the decentralized nature of the US health statistics system, it is hard to obtain a cost figure for the total health statistics effort. However, expenditures for the major, general-purpose statistical efforts are shown in Figure 8.6. Approximately 50 per cent of the total health statistics budget for the agencies shown is spent on collecting and analyzing health status data. The proportion of the various agencies budgets spent for health status varies from over 95 per cent by the Center for Disease Control (CDC) to 1.6 per cent spent by the Health Resources Administration (HRA). The ranges spent on resource and utilization data are similar but the highs and lows are observed for different agencies; this reflects the different missions of these governmental units.

Future Directions

The US as a model. The similar experiences in Europe and the United States with regard to the rising costs for health care and the increasing demands for health service would indicate that the US health statistics might well serve as a useful model. Since the problems that the decision makers face are similar, it is reasonable that they might both benefit from the same data. However, in using the US as a model, it is important to realize that there are cultural differences between the US and various European nations. Thus, while the US health indicator information system can serve as a model, these differences must be considered in selecting the specific elements and indicators for European health information systems.

As shown in figure 8.6, the cost of collecting these data is not trivial. Thus, analysis of the strengths of existing health data systems by national policy makers can pinpoint not only the data to be collected, but also the possible economies in this collection. Due to the extensive amount of data available in, and on, the US health statistics system, this single source provides European policy makers with information for making a cost-benefit analysis for having their own health statistics system.

Gaps in Current Health Indicator Information Systems. Health indicator information systems have gaps in subject matter that may be specific for national policy. An example of this in the US health statistics system is the small amount of health status data available on minorities, for example the Hispanics. The focus of public policy on Hispanics has resulted in the modification of the National Health and Nutrition Examination Survey (NHANES) to obtain information on this minority group.[14] Apart from more knowledge about certain minorities and high risk groups, the following priorities in future health statistics are to be found: (1) more indicators of programme effectiveness; (2) more knowledge about high risk groups in the population; (3) more knowledge in the monitoring and assessment of the quality of medical care; (4) development of a regional hospital discharge abstract system; (5) more information about ambulatory care; and (6) more information on consumer satisfaction with health services.

Within the input-output approach described above, the process of political decision making in health care could also be assessed. Extension of the indicator systems to include data on the behaviour of decision makers is important in all countries and particularly in highly federalized nations. This would be a major step in the direction of developing a consistent national health policy. The creation of a centralized, multipurpose health statistics system could be an indispensable prerequisite for a national health policy and for research purposes.

Of the health status variables assessed in the health data systems above, only those of perceived health status and well-being attempt to measure the positive side of health. The other health status variables measure and assess the level of disease, disability and death in a community. With their emphasis on the negative side of health, they are proxies of health status. Like the perceived health status variable, the accuracy of these proxies in assessing health status needs further research. Also, it is possible that indicators in the existing health information systems can be scaled to create on overall health index.

Cross-national comparisons. International comparisons of health data have always been useful in setting health policies. The adoption of a common framework, prospectively, should facilitate the comparability of data. In setting up such an information system, the framework should be flexible to allow for data to cover specific, unique intranational health concerns as well as to allow for a core of data to be collected by a group of nations for international comparisons. One advantage of using the US health indicator information system as a model is that this would allow for comparisons with US health conditions as well as within the cooperating European nations.

NOTES

1. Occasionally the key functions of health statistics are grouped as to: (a) resource allocation (selecting priorities, projecting problems and needs): (b) evaluation (programme evaluation): (c) comparison (monitoring trends, social indicators).

   For more details and examples, see for example Woolsey 1975 and Berg 1973. For more recent information see Chapter 8 *Health Statistics in Office of Federal Statistical Policy and Standards* (in date), see also in regard to the construction, use and application of health indicators, Culyer, *et al.* 1972, 94–103 and Jazairi 1976, 12–21.

2. See, for example, *Department of Health Education and Welfare 1976*, 129–170, and the current issues of the *Statistical Notes for Health Planners*, published by the National Center for Health Statistics, Hyattsville, Maryland.

3. Fuchs (1979). With regard to the value of health statistics, one could argue that they are a prerequisite for proving the highly controversial opinion that health care doesn't matter. For a systematic discussion of the importance of indicators, with special reference to health indicators, for social policy, see Henke 1975.

4. For a proposal to group the health indicators according to the human life cycle, see Jazairi 1976. See also the *National Center for Health Statistics 1977*.

5. A glance at the contents of statistical publications on health care confirm many of the different health care levels that were used in figure 8.1. See for example *National Center for Health Statistics 1979, Department of Health Education and Welfare 1979, Organization for Economic Cooperation and Development 1977* and *OECD*, Henke 1977, 20–79.

6. Ongoing surveys are collected at regular intervals and are of general interest whereas special or one-time surveys are designed to provide insight into a topical issue. A summary of some of the US health statistics information systems is given in *Office of Technology Assessment 1979*, 11.

7. In 1974, the US Congress mandated that health data collected from the various sources be compiled and presented to members of Congress annually. This compendium provides the legislators with a statement about the health of the population, its use of services, and the amount of resources and expenditures of the delivery system, as well as providing detailed analysis of selected health concerns. This 1979 report to Congress illustrates how

health data which are provided to the policy makers fit the proposed framework. The detailed chapters are: Health Status of Minority Groups; Diet, Nutrition, Disease and the Dietary Goals; Current Status and Future Prospects of Nonphysician Health Care Providers; and, Medical Technology Assessment, Greater Research Community Involvement. These chapter headings are in *Health US 1979*, (National Center for Health Statistics 1979, ix–x).

8. These examples of disaggregation have been taken from Tables 24 and 144 of *Health US 1979* and *Health US 1978*, published by the National Center for Health Statistics, Hyattsville, Maryland. The *Current Listing* and *Topical Index*, also available from the National Center for Health Statistics, provides a useful summary of data available from NCHS surveys and of studies of this data analyzed by demographic and socioeconomic variables.

9. For a discussion of the functions of the health statistics collection and analysis efforts in DHHS, the reader is referred to *Department of Health Education and Welfare 1979*. This volume is issued annually by DHHS and highlights current activities as well as directions for the near future. One of the principal concerns of the most recent issue is the ability to coordinate between the various health data collection agencies.

10. The use of health statistics is outlined in *Office of Technology Assessment 1979*, 10.

11. Summaries of the agencies, their functions and organizational affiliations, are presented in *Selected Topics in Federal Health Statistics*, ibid., p. 3, and *Health Statistics Plan Fiscal Years 1979–1980*, pp. 14–19.

12. Information about the design of the various surveys conducted by NCHS is published in *Vital and Health Statistics*. Series 1 Number 2 describes the design of the National Health Interview Survey; a summary of questionnaires used from 1954 to 1974 is available in Series 1, Number 11. The National Health Examination Survey is described in Series 1 Number 4; the update of this survey to include the measurement of nutrition, the National Health and Nutrition Examination Survey, is described in Series 1, Number 10, parts A and B. Information about health facilities data collection system is presented in Series 1, Numbers 3 and 6. More recent surveys, the National Survey of Nursing Homes and the Master Facility Inventory Survey are presented in Series 1, Numbers 7 and 9, respectively, and the National Ambulatory Medical Care Survey, in Series 2, Number 61.

13. Additional information about the scope and services of the Clearinghouse on Health Indices is available in each issue of the *Bibliography on Health Indexes*. To receive information from the Clearinghouse, write to Ms. Pennifer Erickson, Clearinghouse on Health Indices, Division of Environmental Epidemiology, Office of Analysis and Epidemiology Program: MCHS: DHHS, Center Building, Room 2–27, 3700 East-West Highway, Hyattsville, MD 20782, USA.

14. This survey is currently in the design and pretest stage. The National Center for Health Statistics expects data collection for the main survey to begin in mid-1981.

APPENDIX A: GLOSSARY OF ACRONYMS FOR THE US HEALTH INFORMATION SYSTEM

ADAMHA	Alcohol, Drug Abuse, and Mental Health Administration
BCHS	Bureau of Community Health Services
BD	Bureau of Drugs
BHE	Bureau of Health Education
BHF	Bureau of Health Facilities Financing, Compliance, and Conversion
BHM	Bureau of Health Manpower
BHP	Bureau of Health Planning
BLS	Bureau of Labor Statistics
BMD	Bureau of Medical Devices
BMS	Bureau of Medical Services
BRH	Bureau of Radiological Health
CDC	Centers for Disease Control
CPSC	Consumer Product Safety Commission
EPA	Environmental Protection Agency
ESRD	End-Stage Renal Disease
FDA	Food and Drug Administration
HCFA	Health Care Financing Administration
HDAC	Health Data Advisory Committee
HRA	Health Resources Administration
HSA	Health Services Administration
HSCC	Health Statistics Coordinating Committee
IHS	Indian Health Service
MESA	Mining Enforcement and Safety Administration
NCHCT	National Center for Health Care Technology
NCHS	National Center for Health Statistics
NCHSR	National Center for Health Services Research
NCI	National Cancer Institute
NCVHS	National Committee on Vital and Health Statistics
NHLBI	National Heart, Lung, and Blood Institute
NHTSA	National Highway Traffic Safety Administration
NIAAA	National Institute on Alcohol Abuse and Alcoholism
NICHD	National Institute of Child Health and Human Development
NIDA	National Institute on Drug Abuse
NIH	National Institute of Health
NIMH	National Institute of Mental Health
NINCDS	National Institute of Neurological and Communicative Disorders and Stoke
NIOSH	National Institute of Occupational Safety and Health
OASH	Office of the Assistant Secretary for Health
OASPE	Office of the Assistant Secretary for Planning and Evaluation
OFSPS	Office of Federal Statistical Policy and Standards
OHDS	Office of Human Development
OHMO	Office of Health Maintenance Organizations

OHRST	Office of Health Research, Statistics, and Technology
OPE	Office of Planning and Evaluation
OPPR	Office of Policy, Planning, and Research
ORDS	Office of Research, Demonstrations and Statistics
OSHA	Occupational Safety and Health Administration
OSP	Office of Statistical Policy
PHS	Public Health Service
PSRO	Professional Standards Review Organization
VA	Veterans Administration

APPENDIX B: SUMMARIES OF MAJOR ACTIVITIES OF STATISTICAL AGENCIES
IN THE US DEPARTMENT OF HEALTH AND HUMAN SERVICES (DHHS)

Office of the Assistant Secretary for Planning and Evaluation (OASPE)

The Assistant Secretary for Planning and Evaluation (ASPE), DHHS, serves as the principal adviser to the Secretary of DHHS on appropriate economic, social and programme analysis matters and is responsible for coordinating the forward planning activities of the Department, which encompass formulating and analyzing alternative legislative proposals, policy analysis, and research and evaluation planning. This mission is accomplished through an organization consisting of functional and programmatic units, an approach which provides both an operational framework to direct, coordinate, and evaluate certain departmental activities, and a research and analytic capability to perform policy analyses.

Within OASPE, the Office of Planning and Evaluation/Health (OPE/H) is the principal office which directly interfaces with the Department's health agencies to coordinate the health-related issues of the planning, policy analysis, and legislative formulation process and which conducts research, analyses, and evaluation activities in the health area. OPE/H is organized into divisions of Health Financing and Cost Analysis, Health Evaluation and Prevention Programs, and Health Resources and Services. In addition to its Health Component, OASPE includes a Division of Statistics which participates in the following activities: technical coordination of selected cross-cutting statistical activities within the Department, representation of the Department in dealing with other Federal agencies on matters of statistical data collection, establishment of congruent definitions and classifications for statistics of departmental concern, performance of special studies and research to improve existing statistical techniques, and planning and coordination of major data collections to acquire data for policy analysis and evaluation.

Health Care Financing Administration (HCFA)

As the agency responsible for the Federal government's two major health care financing programmes (Medicare and Medicaid), NCFA maintains large data files describing Federal health care expenditures, health care providers, and HCFA programme beneficiaries.

Medicare programme statistics are maintained centrally on a person level basis. Linkages are made across beneficiary, claims and provider information. Medicaid programme statistics at the Federal level are aggregate and do not allow for person based linkages and analyses. The majority of these data are produced as a direct result of bill processing and related support systems established to reimburse providers of health care services under Medicare and Medicaid. The balance of the health data maintained within HCFA is generated through HCFA's quality assurance programs, special research studies, and demonstration and evaluation projects focusing upon various aspects of health care cost-containment and quality assurance.

Most of the research, demonstration, and evaluation responsibility within HCFA is vested in the Office of Research, Demonstrations and Statistics (ORDS). ORDS is also responsible for maintaining various data files generated from Medicare bill processing network and reporting on Medicaid aggregate statistics. HCFA's needs for health data can be divided into four general categories. The first includes data requirements attendant to the provider reimbursement systems, and essentially includes data sets which describe the nature and costs of health care services received by HCFA programme beneficiaries, and identify and describe the beneficiary and the site of these services. These data are used to make payment decisions. The second categorical need for health data relates to HCFA's quality assurance programmes. Under these programmes, data are required to monitor various quality characteristics of health care providers (for example, hospital environmental safety factors). Additionally, health data are needed in this area to support peer review conducted under the auspices of HCFA's Professional Standards Review Organization (PSRO) programme in the form of provider profiles and 'norms' of health care. Programme and project evaluation represent a third category of health data needs. HCFA conducts empirical evaluation studies of the impact of its major programmes and demonstration projects on an ongoing basis. Data for these studies may draw upon one or more of HCFA's operational data systems. The final category of health data needs concern those data required to support research and broad initiatives in the area of cost containment and health care reimbursement reform.

Office of Human Development Services (OHDS)

OHDS is the principal operating component of the Department responsible for human development programmes and social services. Though its five programme administration and three staff units, OHDS administers programmes that serve the following populations: children (disadvantaged, disabled, abused and neglected), handicapped (physical and mental), aged, native americans, low income adults and families, and runaway youth.

OHDS acts as an advocate in the department for the special population groups it serves, and develops actions and strategies to improve coordination of human development services within the department, in the federal government, with state and local government, and with private sector organizations. OHDS uses status data on its service populations, and some of those data are 'health' data or statistics. Thus, OHDS' definition of statistics is a broad one.

Elements of the OHDS routine data collection systems which include some health statistics include:

(1) family planning, information and referral, health related services, and home-maker services;
(2) diagnostic services and types of disabling conditions related to vocational rehabilitation;
(3) health screening, nutrition and immunizations for children;
(4) diagnosis, treatment and health planning related to developmental disabilities;
(5) alcohol and drug abuse, venereal diseases, and pregnancies in adolescents.

Public Health Service (PHS)

PHS is the principal health agency of the Federal Government. Its mission, in its broadest and simplest terms, is to protect and advance the health of the American people. Health data activities of the Public Health Service, both general purpose and programme-specific, support this mission. Because of their diversity, major organizational units of the PHS are described separately below.

Alcohol, Drug Abuse and Mental Health Administration (ADAMHA) has responsibility for national research, training and services in the areas of alcoholism, drug abuse and mental illness. Its three component agencies, the National Institute of Mental Health (NIMH), the National Institute on Alcohol Abuse and Alcoholism (NIAAA), and the National Institute on Drug Abuse (NIDA), each engage in a number of significant statistical activities directed at identifying the location and characteristics of facilities, programmes and personnel providing services to their target population; counting the numbers and characteristics of persons served by their programme funds; determining charges and sources of payment for services; and assessing the effectiveness of services provided. While the statistical activities of each Institute are specifically tailored to serve its particular programme needs, an overall ADANHA Data Coordinating Committee is continuing to work toward the development of common definitions and categories for patient, facility and staff variables.

Centers for Disease Control (CDC) is the Federal Government's focal point for the prevention and control of preventable diseases, laboratory improvement, health education and occupational safety and health. CDC's overall mission is to monitor disease patterns and to provide assistance to state, local and other health related institutions in controlling disease and preventing its reoccurrence. As the incidence of known communicable disease has declined, CDC's programmes have been expanded to include noncommunicable but preventable diseases, including dental diseases. Data are collected and published weekly on the incidence of hepatitis, botulism, tuberculosis, venereal diseases, etc. CDC provides project grants to state and local health agencies for immunization, prevention and control of childhood lead-based paint poisoning, venereal diseases control, and urban rat control. CDC also carries out regulatory activities, such as monitoring of laboratory standards, occupational health hazard evaluation, and prevention of disease importation from other countries.

Food and Drug Administration (FDA) is a regulatory agency whose mission is consumer protection in certain areas of health. FDA plays a significant role in influencing the nation's health status and in assuring the effectiveness of the nation's health care delivery system by ensuring that: (1) food is safe and wholesome, (2) drugs, biological products, therapeutic devices, and diagnostic products are safe and effective, (3) cosmetics are safe, (4) the use of radiological products does not result in unnecessary exposure to radiation, and (5) all of these products are honestly labelled. In addition, FDA engages in special studies dealing with nutrition education and knowledge, food additives usage, perceptions concerning products labelling and patient-packet inserts, adverse reactions to cosmetics, and prescription drug advertising.

Health Resources Administration (HRA) is responsible for identifying health care resource problems and maintaining or strengthening the distribution, supply, use, quality and cost-effectiveness of these resources in order to improve the health care systems and the health status of individual members of the population. In order to carry out its mission effectively, HPA requires extensive data on the health status of the population, the accessibility to and use of health care services, and measures of the Nation's health planning and resource development capacities, especially its manpower production capacity.

Health Services Administration (HSA) has responsibility for those programmes of the PHS that deal with direct service delivery to statutory beneficiaries, building the primary care capacity for medically underserved populations, and for assuring quality in federally financed health care services. Direct health care services are provided in PHS facilities and with PHS employees, to American Indians and Alaska natives and to merchant seamen and other designated beneficiaries. Some care for these individuals is also provided through contract and formula grants to public and non-profit organizations for building primary care capacity where medical care access is limited. Other capacity building programmes include Emergency Medical Services Systems (EMSS). Therefore, the data needs of the HSA programmes differ widely, ranging from detailed medical history and clinical data aggregated by patient to summary information on the services provided by grantees.

National Institutes of Health (NIH) is the leading Federal agency for biomedical research concerning the prevention, diagnosis, and treatment of disease. The management of such an enterprise involves a wide variety of data. One type of data focuses on the incidence, prevalence, and cost of disease in the country required for the establishment of priorities in the investment of public funds and

allocation of limited resources for the research effort. Another type is epidemiological data which provide non-laboratory statistics for testing hypotheses
relating to disease states and conditions and are important in complementing the
search for the etiology and pathogenesis of diseases. A concerted effort is under-
way in NIH to review and identify common needs for data of this sort in the
various Institutes and Offices of the NIH in order to ensure that the limited
funds for such statistical and analytical activities are used in the most efficient
and effective manner.

Office of the Assistant Secretary for Health (OASH). The Office of Health
Research, Statistics and Technology (OHRST) is the principal office within
OASH concerned with health statistics. OHRST includes the National Center for
Health Care Technology, the National Center for Health Services Research, and
the National Center for Health Statistics, one of the five major, general purpose
statistical agencies of the Federal government. OHRST not only strengthens the
Department's capability to stimulate and assess technological developments in
health and apply the latest technologies to medical practice, but strengthens the
relationship among technology assessment, health services research, and health
statistics as a basis for health policy formulation.

Material in this appendix has been adopted from *Health Statistics Plan*, Fiscal
Years 1979–1980, (DHEW 1979).

9

Health Monitoring
in England and Wales

A J FOX

With the systematic collection and regular analysis of many of its current statistics on health going back to the pioneering works of Farr, Guy, Chadwick and Nightingale in the early 19th century, England and Wales are fortunate in having a reasonably well-developed health information system that enables administrators and researchers to study different aspects of the health of the nation. This paper outlines the need for health data, what data are routinely collected, how they are used to monitor the health of the population and how they can be related to environmental changes.

THE NEED FOR DATA

In the last century, when death rates particularly for infants, children and young adults were so much higher than they are today, medical and social scientists were concerned to demonstrate the relationships between health and the circumstances in which people lived. It was clear from relatively simple studies of the causes of death and their different distribution among various subgroups of the population that the effects of many of the diseases that lead to death would be minimised by improvements in sanitation, hygiene and diet. Improvements took place and, as a direct consequence, the infectious diseases which took such a heavy toll of deaths in the last century have almost disappeared (McKeown 1976). These diseases have now been replaced by the modern epidemics of heart disease, accidents and cancers (Office of Population Censuses and Surveys 1978). These are not infectious diseases in the sense that they spread from individual to individual but only in the sense that the social environment and behaviour which leads to their increase spreads from social group to social group.

Despite the considerable impetus given to the collection of hospital statistics by Florence Nightingale (Cullen 1975) mortality statistics have continued to provide the main platform of national health data. The death certificate, even with its limitations in terms of recording diseases and history leading to death, can still be a more reliable and interpretable indicator of health than are morbidity records. It is not surprising, therefore, that the Department of Health and Social Security when attempting to allocate resources on the basis of health 'need' turns to mortality indicators to measure that need (Department of Health and Social Security 1976). Nevertheless, as will be clear from the next section, morbidity data are now widely collected and used to monitor health.

In the new environment of risk assessment the Royal Society points to five main reasons for collecting epidemiological observations on man (Royal Society 1983). These are:

(1)   man's behaviour and way of life;
(2)   the inadequacy of animal models:
(3)   the need to study dose—response relationships and thresholds;
(4)   the need to monitor environmental control; and
(5)   the study of disease progression.

Many of the hazards to which man is exposed reflect his behaviour and way of life. In particular, the hazards of hang-gliding, motor cycling and mountain climbing could not be properly assessed without systematic records of accidents being maintained.

While it is becoming increasingly important to study the response of animals to potential toxic or carcinogenic chemicals it is recognized by most toxicologists that the animal model may not provide a reliable predictor of man's reaction to exposure to the same materials. Man may react differently because of his genetic constitution or because of behavioural differences in particular in terms of diet and social behaviour. Also animals may not reliably predict morbidity effects that, though less severe than mortality, may be very important.

The limitations of animal models are even greater when it comes to decisions about environmental control and the need to estimate the dose—response relationships and to predict the thresholds above which man will react. It is now recognised that moves to larger and larger animal experiments (the mega-mouse experiment) may not be the most appropriate way of tackling these questions and the Royal Society suggests that controlled, monitored release of new substances should provide adequate safeguards (Royal Society 1983).

It has also been recognized for many years that even where good scientific evidence exists there is a need to monitor health in order to identify those hazards to man that were not predicted on the basis of animal or other tests and to indicate those areas where environmental control of previously recognized hazards has proved unsatisfactory. This continuous evaluation of hazards becomes a central aspect of risk management of new exposures as well as of old hazards (Royal Society 1983).

While the most direct approach to disease prevention may be through the control of exposure the medical profession has recognised that such social engineering is not always possible and that one of its main functions is to study disease development and progression in order to identify stages at which the individual can be cured or further progress can be prevented. Recognition of the important role of the medical profession in screening and cure emphasises the need for proper morbidity statistics to help evaluate the contribution of the medical profession to improvements in health. Only studies separating differentials in disease incidence from subsequent survival provide a proper evaluation of the impact of medical intervention (Office of Population Censuses and Surveys 1980).

ROUTINE COLLECTION OF HEALTH DATA

Most routine health data for England and Wales are collected for or by government departments according to their responsibility to subgroups of the population. It should be recognised however that national records are often reduced in quality to the level of the least co-operative contributor and that local records for some aspects of health will be more reliable and more detailed. The national cancer registration scheme is an example where analysis and follow-up based on local data may prove more fruitful than analysis of national data. Nevertheless national data are needed to provide an overall perspective on health.

For a detailed review of national health statistics the reader is referred to Alderson and Whitehead (1974) and to the proceedings of the 1980 Statistics Users' Conference (Health Statistics in Britain, forthcoming). The main government departments collecting or co-ordinating health data are the Office of Population Censuses and Surveys (OPCS), the Department of Health and Social Security (DHSS), the Public Health Laboratory Service (PHLS), Communicable Disease Surveillance Centre, the Employment Medical Advisory Service (EMAS), which is part of the Health and Safety Executive and the Department of Education and Science (DES). The data collected by these departments concern the population as a whole (or large sub-sets) but the Civil Service Department and the Ministry of Defence also collect records about the health of their employees.

Historically, national health data were first collected by the General Register Office which analysed vital registration records on births, deaths and marriages. Since 1970, this function has been combined with that of the Government Social Survey, who were responsible for ad hoc surveys, in the OPCS (Redfern 1976). The new organization is now involved in the collection and publication of birth and death statistics, hospital statistics from the Hospital In-patient Enquiry (HIPE), cancer registration and survival statistics, statistics on abortions and on congenital malformations as well as statistics on notified infectious diseases. The Office is also involved with a number of ad hoc studies such as the National Morbidity Survey which has looked at morbidity in select general practices and regular sample surveys such as the General Household Survey, a random population sample survey which includes general health questions.

As well as co-ordinating the Hospital Activity Analysis, the DHSS collects data through the Mental Health Enquiry which covers all in-patients receiving NHS phychiatric care and through registration of disabled persons, sickness benefit claims and other benefit claims such as for industrial diseases and injuries.

The PHLS is responsible for following up local outbreaks of disease which may have a common environmental origin. These follow-ups are used to compile Communicable Disease Reports.

EMAS also collects much information through its own field force of about one hundred doctors. This generally falls under two head-ings; the first covering statutory periodic medical examinations of groups such as lead workers, the second describes the data collected in routine or ad hoc surveys such as the national survey of asbestos workers. At the same time the Health and Safety at Work etc Act (1974) places responsibility on employers to be aware of any work-related health effects on their employees.

The final government department in the above list was the DES which is responsible for the health of school children under the 1944 Education Act and collects the results of regular examinations of all school children.

As already indicated above the reader who is interested in a more detailed account of national health records should refer to Alderson and Whitehead (1974).

MONITORING HEALTH TRENDS

One reason why systematic health data are collected is that they enable various groups to detect patterns and unexpected deviations in disease and disease trends for which an explanation should be sought. A number of approaches to monitoring trends have been developed, some rely heavily on the formal regular analysis of the statistical data, others benefit more from the development of highly motivated clinically aware members of the medical profession.

It is important to recognize that in the past the latter group, who are after all directly involved with patients, have been responsible for the detection of many 'epidemics'. They have identified changing patterns of a disease through their clinical awareness rather than through formal monitoring systems. However even in such examples it has often proved necessary to turn to routine records in order to evaluate their hypotheses. An example is the discovery of the high nasal cancer rate in High Wycombe associated with work in the furniture industry (Acheson *et al.* 1968). This example is interesting because the formal follow-up study, as well as confirming the initial hypothesis, also identified a second problem in the boot and shoe industry (Acheson *et al.* 1972).

Given the number of initial hypotheses on the causation of disease that are being generated from within the medical profession it is useful for a country to develop a system of bringing these together. An example of a relatively simple idea which has been developed in the field of drug testing is the DHSS Yellow Card System. The DHSS Committee on Safety in Medicines asks medical practitioners to report on a yellow card all reactions to recently introduced drugs as well as serious or unusual reactions to other drugs, including vaccines. As a result of the information received the Committee may publish a warning in the 'Adverse Reactions Series', or under 'Current Problems' if further studies are needed before a definitive statement is possible. There are other examples of how the development of local networks can improve monitoring and increase the likelihood of detecting problems earlier (Inman 1981a and b).

The above monitoring is based mainly on the medical profession with the statistics providing support. The last ten years or so has seen, in particular within OPCS, the application of statistical techniques for detecting significant trends or deviations in the routine health statistics OPCS collects. These tests are now routinely applied to mortality data (OPCS 1981) (annually), to congenital malformation data (Weatherall 1978) (monthly and quarterly tests by area are reported to Area Medical Officers) and to infectious disease data (Goldblatt, no date) (fortnightly tests by area reported to DHSS). In addition OPCS is planning to apply similar tests to hospital in patient data from HIPE.

Health data collected by these government agencies are also analysed and reviewed at regular intervals. As well as publishing over forty reports in its series on studies in medical and population subjects (for example Heady and Heasman 1959) the OPCS has a long history of decennial supplements on mortality which goes back to 1841 (OPCS 1978). These reviews which look in depth at mortality by area, occupation and cause of death have recently been supplemented by data being collected in the OPCS Longitudinal Study which permits the analysis of mortality by the full range of census characteristics (Fox and Goldblatt 1982).

TRENDS IN ENVIRONMENT

Whereas environmental factors in health were widely recognised in the last century there was a period at the beginning of this century when it was thought that the new diseases, the cancers and circulatory diseases, reflected genetic factors and differences in 'ageing'. It is now widely accepted that the process of ageing is strongly influenced by environment in the broadest sense. People are exposed to environmental hazards at work, through personal habits and way of life as well as in their area of residence.

Many organizations are responsible for measuring substances in the environment to assess present levels and to predict future trends. For example, the National Survey on Air Pollution has been monitoring air pollutants for the last 20 years, following the Clean Air Act (1956). Reorganization of the water industry in 1974 brought into being the Water Research Centre whose Medmenham laboratories are particularly concerned with water quality in relation to health. In 1965 the Natural Environmental Research Council was established and it supports research on air pollution by sulphur and nitrogen oxides, marine pollution by radioactive waste, and freshwater pollution by fertilisers, trace metals and pesticides. The Department of the Environment (Central Unit for Environmental Pollution), the Ministry of Agriculture, Fisheries and Food and the Monitoring and Assessment Research Centre are all actively involved in measuring environmental pollutions.

Similarly the Health and Safety at Work etc. Act (1974) ensures that the occupational environment is subject to a certain degree of monitoring. In particular the Health and Safety Executive (HSE) has specified limits for chemical substances, mineral dust and nuisance particulates in workroom air and has established a system whereby the use of new potentially toxic substances is routinely reported to HSE. Recent discussion documents have also suggested the proper maintenance of personnel and other records for health monitoring.

The personal environment has been more difficult to monitor systematically and for data in this area epidemiologists generally turn to the general surveys conducted by the Government Statistical Service. Such surveys would include in particular the National Food Survey, the General Household Survey and the Family Expenditure Survey. The lack of adequate data on cigarette consumption before 1950 illustrates the problem of relying on these sources; nevertheless they have proved of considerable value in population-based correlation studies.

POPULATION-BASED CORRELATION STUDIES

As was suggested above one of the important roles of population health statistics and population environment statistics is that they can be used at the aggregate level to correlate health and environment. Historically this has been the most popular way of analyzing these data because such data are relatively simple to collect, either because routine administrative systems are expected to produce the relevant statistics or because data can be derived on a sample basis.

Population-based correlation studies have generally looked at time trends, geographic (international as well as regional) and occupational differences. Concentration on these characteristics primarily reflects their systematic recording on most routine health records.

Studies have shown that the rising tide of drunkeness offences, hospital admissions and deaths due to alcoholism parallel the increase in alcohol consumption since the Second World War (Donnan and Haskey 1977). Trends in sales and prescriptions of pressurised aerosols and deaths from asthma, strongly suggested that misuse of these dispensers was responsible for the increased mortality among young people in the 1960s (Inman and Adelstein 1969). Associations between unusually cold weather and short-term increases in mortality, particularly from ischaemic heart disease have been noted (Rose 1966), but, with the decline in concentrations of suspended particulates pollutants, the association seen in the 1950s and early

1960s between daily mortality and air pollution is no longer apparent (McFarlane 1977).

Comparisons of mortality differentials between countries clearly demonstrated the association between mortality from arteriosclerotic heart disease and lung cancer in relation to national levels of smoking (Reid 1975). More recently the approach has been used to relate cardiovascular disease mortality to trends in oral contraception use (Beral 1976).

Within England and Wales studies of differences in mortality by county borough have suggested a strong association between cardiovascular mortality and soft drinking water (Crawford *et al.* 1971) and have indicated the effect of high air pollution on the prevalence of bronchitis and ear disease (Reid 1969). Similarly, occupational differences in cigarette consumption have also been related to lung cancer mortality using data from the General Household Survey and the latest Decennial Supplement (Fox 1977).

It should be recognized that the evidence provided by population-based correlation studies is circumstantial. Although an association between disease and some factor may be revealed, the interpretation may be obscured by relationships with other factors that have not been measured but which may be the underlying cause of the disease in question. However although an association may not provide definitive evidence of causation, it does point to possible risk factors and to communities where further study of individuals would be worthwhile.

INDIVIDUAL-BASED STUDIES

Recent developments in cancer and mortality statistics in England and Wales have led to a large increase in the number of individual-based studies which contrast the health of a group of people, all of whom had been individually exposed to the substances in question, with that of a group none of whom have been exposed. Such studies, which make use of the National Health Service Central Register at Southport to obtain copies of cancer and mortality records for the individuals being followed, are now widely used to answer questions about health of particular occupational groups (Fox 1981b) or groups who were exposed to suspect compounds during the course of medical treatment. The recent study of the mortality of ankylosing spondilitics is an example of the latter approach being used to assess the health effects of radiation exposure (Court-Brown and Doll 1965).

Studies concentrating on occupational groups or people who have been medically treated are important because quite often these groups are found to have been exposed to high concentrations of suspect materials and because, in well-designed studies, detailed exposure histories allow the epidemiologist to allow for confounding factors in his analysis. Also, the substances to which occupational groups are exposed may be those to which the public are exposed at lower levels. The EMAS studies of asbestos and lead workers were intended to estimate the risks to the population at large as well as those faced by these particular groups.

Studies of migrant populations, who commonly change behaviour as well as environment when they migrate, and studies of other well defined groups of individuals, have proved important in assessing the relationship between environment and health. The classic study of doctors illustrates how a questionnaire approach linked to subsequent mortality was used by Doll and Hill (1964) to show the empirical support for hypotheses about the effects of cigarette smoking.

The OPCS Longitudinal Study indicates how routine record linkage between administrative records can be used to improve the understanding of morbidity and mortality differentials. Record linkage means that the scope of statistics is considerably broadened and that the time relationships between exposures and effects can be studied. The OPCS Longitudinal Study has already been used to indicate the marked differentials between social groups characterised by housing circumstances and, by looking at the mortality of regional migrants, to show that regional differentials in mortality are not a consequence of migration patterns between the regions (Fox 1980). The time discussion has been used to develop a theory indicating how selection affects mortality differentials and thereby to evaluate the effects of selection on occupational differences, geographic differences, and marital status differences as well as on the differences by household circumstances (Fox 1981a).

The main problem with these individual based studies is that, unless the epidemiologist is able to find a suitable cohort that many years earlier was subject to the environment in question, the follow-up period is necessarily long. After all, for the main diseases, in which interest lies, mortality will only occur a number of years after the relevant exposure. As these studies involve the acquisition and follow-up of individuals' records they are necessarily more expensive than population-based correlation studies.

USERS

Health statistics are needed in local practice and hospitals for patient management to identify problems as well as to allay suspicions of epidemics. They are also needed for the local management of health services. At the regional or national level they are needed to monitor the health of the nation and to afford researchers the opportunity to follow-up clues that may be emanating from local investigation. In the latter context, the Medical Research Council, individual universities and individual government departments are well represented in the attached appendix which lists units who in recent years made extensive use of national statistics in the study of disease aetiology. The recent establishment of the Epidemiological Monitoring Unit at the London School of Hygiene and Tropical Medicine, and the MRC Environmental Epidemiology Unit at Southampton University are ample reflection of the growing belief in the potential of routine health data subjected to systematic analysis. The achievements of these units over the next few years should serve to emphasize the role of routine data collection in monitoring, and hence to improving, the health of the nation.

APPENDIX: USERS OF ROUTINE HEALTH STATISTICS IN THE STUDY
OF ENVIRONMENTAL HEALTH PROBLEMS

The following are some examples of MRC units, university departments, government departments and other organizations which use routine health data in monitoring disease and health care.

Epidemiological Monitoring Unit, Department of Medical Statistics and Epidemiology, and Department of Community Health, London School of Hygiene and Tropical Medicine.
Division of Epidemiology, Institute of Cancer Research, Sutton.
Department of Regius Professor of Medicine, Oxford.
Department of Social and Community Medicine, Oxford.
Cancer Epidemiology and Clinical Trials Unit, Oxford.
Children's Cancer Research Group, Oxford.
Department of Community Medicine, University of Southampton.
Department of Clinical Epidemiology and Social Medicine, St. George's Hospital, London.
Department of Social Medicine, St. Thomas's Hospital, London.
Department of Clinical Epidemiology and Social Medicine, Royal Free Hospital, London.

TUC Centenary Institute of Occupational Medicine, London School of Hygiene and Tropical Medicine.

Department of Occupational Health and Safety, Aston University, Birmingham.

Social Statistics Research Unit, Department of Mathematics, City University, London.

MRC Epidemiology and Medical Care Unit, Northwick Park Hospital.

MRC Environmental Hazards Unit, St. Bartholomew's Hospital, London.

MRC Epidemiology Unit (South Wales), Cardiff.

MRC Environmental Epidemiology Unit, Southampton General Hospital, Coxford Road, Southampton.

MRC Pneumoconiosis Research Unit, Penarth.

MRC Toxiology Unit, Carshalton.

Medical Statistics Division, Office of Population Censuses and Surveys.

Communicable Disease Surveillance Centre, Public Health Laboratory Service, Colindale.

Birmingham and West Midlands Regional Cancer Registry, Birmingham.

Employment Medical Advisory Service (Health and Safety Executive).

Institute of Occupational Medicine, Edinburgh.

10

Disability as a Health Indicator

RORY WILLIAMS

INTRODUCTION

Disability assessments now serve an increasing number of uses: they are not only an aspect of diagnosis and prognosis in individual cases, but they also may measure the outcome of treatment for varying diagnoses in groups that experience different treatments, different placements, or different allocations of resources. Again, where improvements through treatment are not expected, disability assessments may be used to estimate the relative disadvantage of individuals or groups of patients, or to account for the demands on resources which they make. As all these uses have developed, so the method of measuring disability has had to take into account more and more of the factors affecting the social value placed on disabilities, and in doing so it has had to draw increasingly on the theory of the social sciences. This emphasis on the social, as opposed to the clinical, component of disability is reflected in the definition adopted in this paper, which refers to the disadvantages incurred when specific activities, directed to the purposes of daily life, are restricted in response to a medical condition. This usage corresponds to what Harris (1971) and others (Jefferys *et al.* 1969, WHO 1980) have described as handicap, but, as Harris observed, it is often easier in ordinary speech to use the term disability as I do here.

Disability assessment is a matter of social perceptions and social values in at least three ways. First, disability is only one aspect of a wider social definition of ill health, and its relation to other aspects like the risk of death or the experience of symptoms needs consideration. Secondly disability, as a set of restrictions on normal social activities, is itself a complex phenomenon creating a question about the range of activities which ought to be taken into account. Thirdly, the complex disabilities thus revealed are given varying social values, so that a question arises about how we arrive at a scale of values on which to assess them. The first two questions receive only a brief comment in the next sections, since the reader can refer elsewhere for appropriate discussions, and I concentrate in the rest of the paper on the third question concerning the scale of values assigned to disability, in which some unique possibilities of disability assessment deserve emphasis.

THE RELATION OF DISABILITY TO OTHER HEALTH INDICATORS

Surprisingly little has been done to show the place of disability among other health indicators. Its relation to risk of death on the other hand, and to subjective symptoms of pain, anxiety, depression or tiredness on the other, is still far from certain. The growing popularity of disability measures, in comparison with these other dimensions, is thus largely accounted for by practical considerations: by the limited value of mortality as a health indicator in chronic or degenerative disease, and by the frequent difficulty of obtaining measures of subjective symptoms which are not merely categoric but graduated in a reliable fashion. It might be argued, too, that subjective distress and risk of death are often reflected in restricted activity (Johnson 1972) and where this is the case disability measures become an overall health indicator of great usefulness and practicality. But this argument needs to be used with discrimination: there are situations in which disability and distress are perceived as radically different dimensions (Rosser & Kind 1978) — although the extent to which inverse relationships between disability and distress happen in practice is more limited (Rosser & Watts 1972) — and there are situations in which disability and mortality vary inversely (Isaacs 1972).

Where disability varies separately from other health indicators, there arises the familiar problem of combining the different dimensions. Since this problem has been dealt with in other chapters in this book I do not dwell on it here. Two kinds of solution may, however, be adopted. The first is to establish trade-offs between the various dimensions by one of the many methods available; but a second solution is also available, to restrict the use of disability measures to conditions in which risk of death and subjective distress either vary little or else covary with disability. It is thus no accident that disability is most commonly used as a health indicator in chronic, degenerative diseases where there is little of the risk of imminent death which is often present in, for example, serious traumas and infections, and where pain and distress seldom occurs quite irrespective of physical activity, as it does in say, cancer.

There is also a neglected aspect of the problem of combining dimensions — the question of what aspects of health constitute a single dimension anyway. Perceptions of unity and variety are not, of course, independent of the development of appropriate concepts for particular purposes; for some clinical decisions, the need for great particularity shapes corresponding perceptions of the irreducible variety of health dimensions, while for some policy decisions the need for generalisation shapes corresponding unities. Disability assessment, as a practice used both clinically and in larger policy decisions, is thus much affected by the question of whether disability is a single dimension, and this question, which affects also the scale of values used in assessment, is taken up later in this paper.

THE RANGE OF ACTIVITIES ASSESSED

If the relation of disability to other health indicators has been too little explored, the range of activities relevant to disability assessment is the subject of too vast and uneven a literature to be usefully summarised here. The range of disabilities assessed, the range of restricted activity considered relevant, has been developed gradually over a long period in response to the need for increased sensitivity and comprehensiveness in evaluating the consequences of impairment. The evolving epidemiological recognition that disabilities are not solely properties of individuals but also of their interaction with the culture in which they live, has been a particularly important product of this increasing sensitivity (Wood and Badley 1978). In exploring these interactions qualitative studies have often led the way (Sainsbury 1970, Blaxter 1976) with quantitative measures of the comparative type implied by the term 'health indicator', following along behind (Sainsbury 1973).

It is sufficient for present purposes to refer the reader interested in the selection of relevant disabilities to recent material on the measures available (WHO 1980, Bond and Carstairs in press, Patrick *et al.* in press, Chen and Bush 1979). Choice between these measures inevitably reflects a balance struck between needs for sensitivity and comprehensiveness on the one hand, and for simplicity, specificity and reproducibility on the other; and in striking the balance the context of use is the main consideration. The variety of contexts is discussed elsewhere in this volume (see especially chapter 5).

THE SCALE OF VALUES USED IN ASSESSMENT

Having outlined the nature of the first two questions which need to be resolved in using disability as a health indicator, I now concentrate on scaling problems in the field of disability, leaving aside the question of which disabilities can or ought to be included in the field, and focusing solely on the scaling of existing items. Within that brief I have been still more specific. I have taken as read a huge field of physician or survey ratings on the grounds that they do not claim to compete with each other over forms of scaling but over the definition of suitable items. I think the authors would set little store by the exact numbers, or the exact ranking, which they apply to these items, regarding them, normally correctly, as good enough for general purposes. I have focused accordingly on studies using evidence specifically to establish the order or degree of importance of different disabilities.

In a full account of rank-ordering or scaling attempts two important approaches or sets of approaches would have to receive much more space than they do here. One approach, common to many studies of health indicators at a general level, has been the use of a panel of judges to perform carefully constructed comparisons of health states. In setting up these comparisons theory has been borrowed from psychology, psychophysics and utility modelling, (Mushkin and Dunlop 1979, Rosser and Kind 1978, Culyer 1978, Patrick 1976, Hunt and McEwen 1980), and the result is an overall assessment not just of disability, but of multiple dimensions of health. Because of the concern for these other dimensions, disability is not usually treated in much detail, but there is no reason why these methods should not be used to scale disabilities by themselves. However, the scales they have produced so far have not shown much similarity even in the overall distribution of magnitudes, and it is possible that the abstract setting in which the judgements are made leads to a good deal of variability.

An alternative approach attempts to reveal preferences from natural behaviour. So far this approach has been furthest developed in valuation of human life (Mooney 1977), but there seems to be no reason why it too should not be used in disability assessment. In this use, however, a crucial question is whose preferences and whose behaviour we consider. It is perhaps easiest to study the preferences of resource allocators, and an example is the well-known study of Rosser and Watts (1972) on court decisions in favour of disabled persons. But expert decisions in this area are always vulnerable to doubts about their relation to the preferences of the disabled 'consumer', and so far little has been done to reveal the preferences of the disabled themselves.

Since other papers have dealt with important aspects of these approaches, I concentrate on a third approach focused especially on the natural behaviour of the disabled: cumulative scaling. The approach has shown fairly consistent results with disability and it is already in use in the research of British health departments, so it seems appropriate to make a critical assessment of its development and use so far. Consequently I will leave aside the two sets of approaches already mentioned until I make some general comparisons at the end between their potential and that of the present approach. Firstly I explain the present method; then I consider how far this method has got, where it should go next, and finally, what this means for the whole field of scaling or valuation of health states.

SCALES TAKING ADVANTAGE OF THE CUMULATIVE NATURE OF DISABILITY

The principle of cumulative scaling is very simple. Its basis lies in the fact that many activities or attitudes are ordered in a sequence, and by establishing the sequence, we can at once say whether a given individual is further on, or less far on, than another, in regard to that sequence. It seems possible that many disabilities may fall into such a sequence. If they do, they should tend to fall into patterns like those shown in figure 10.1, where disabled activities are scored 1 and non-disabled activities 0, and there are four activities, of which D is the first to be disabled.

| | Activity items | | | |
Patterns	A	B	C	D
1	0	0	0	1
2	0	0	1	1
3	0	1	1	1
4	1	1	1	1

FIG 10.1 *Cumulative set of disabilities*

The patterns thus form a sequence from mild to severe disability. If disabled individuals are now scored on items A to D, most of them should fall into one of these four patterns, and for each case that does so we can say unequivocally what rank his overall disability attains in comparison with the others.

However, few sequences are perfect. Measurement error is of course a constant possibility: but other kinds of error may also be expected, and these depend partly on the theoretical reasons for supposing that there is a sequence in the first place. Cases showing an error in the sequence may thus be theoretically important, and an advantage of cumulative scaling is the fact that error cases can also be detected unequivocally. In the four-item example just cited, the error cases are shown in figure 10.2.

A	B	C	D
0	0	1	0
0	1	0	0
1	0	0	0
0	1	0	1
1	0	0	1
0	1	1	0
1	0	1	0
1	1	0	0
1	0	1	1
1	1	0	1
1	1	1	0

FIG 10.2 *Error cases*

Whether a given set of disabilities forms a sequence is a matter to be tested. The procedures for testing this will be found elsewhere (Williams *et al.* 1976, Chilton 1969, Tenhouten 1969) and I leave them aside here. The procedures depend on showing that the proportion and pattern of errors do not exceed conventional bounds which would normally assure the stability and repeatability of the sequence. The assurance depends, though, on the sequence being a hypothesis, and not itself a product of inspecting and sorting potential errors beforehand on the same data. Of course, the best assurance of repeatability is, ultimately, repetition.

Once the sequence is established, the error cases have themselves to be assigned a place in the ranking of severity. The assignment of these cases is not determined uniquely by the scaling procedure. In the four-item example, the assignment is a matter of assimilating each error case to one of the four perfect patterns. There are usually two possible ways of doing this; for instance, the case 0010 might be assimilated either to 0001 or to 0011. The choice between these possibilities will again depend on the theoretical grounds for presupposing that there is a sequence among the disabilities concerned.

What, then, are the theoretical requirements for stating a hypothesis that a sequence or cumulative scale underlies the phenomena of disability? The theory involved may be of the most rudimentary possible kind, extending, in the first instance, only to the intuitive perception of disability as a progressive cumulative pattern of recovery or loss along a single dimension. However, this rudimentary notion is not a clear guide to which disability items are relevant, nor to why error cases, other than measurement errors, might occur, nor to how they should be ranked. Decisions about these questions can be made temporarily by assumption, but to decide them ultimately the theory must suggest causes for the existence of a cumulative and unidimensional pattern in disability; and three possible views of causation have been suggested (Williams 1979). The usual assumptions made to decide these questions are that those activities are relevant which adults learn in childhood to carry out in their own, and which are therefore part of adult identity; that error cases arise partly from unconventional choices by individual disabled people and partly from unusual patterns of impairment; and that error cases should be assigned to the rank with the same number of disabilities. On the basis of present theories about social and physical causation, these assumptions appear roughly correct.

Perhaps as important, though, as indicating where theoretical decisions are required, is to emphasise how their absence alters the use of the scale. The minimum requirement is a hypothesis that there is a cumulative and unidimensional pattern in disability. There could easily, however, be no real hypothesis. One way in which this occurs is through the practice, referred to earlier, of sorting the data beforehand to derive the hypothesis in the first place. A similar transformation can however be achieved another way, by choosing item descriptions which are *logically* cumulative and unidimensional. An example would be the following questions.

(1) Can you walk on your own inside the house?
(2) Can you walk on your own outside the house?
(3) Can you walk on your own in the street?

Where the pattern is logical in this way, the exercise of investigating empirical distributions of the items is reduced to an exercise in validation of the researcher's assumptions — to a test of whether disabled respondents mean the same by words as he does. A validation of this kind sometimes has its uses with less obvious examples than the one just given, but they are not the uses proposed here. The present approach requires, on the contrary, that in the case of activities which we know have no necessary logical connection between them, we can show theoretical reasons for expecting them to become disabled fairly uniformly in one cumulative sequence. This sequence can then be subjected to empirical tests.

An emphasis on the theoretical requirements for a scale of handicap, even when the theory is a simple one, has a further importance in suggesting the possibility that some disabilities may cumulate on more than one dimension, and that some may be unidimensional without being cumulative. More than one dimension may be represented when different sub-cultures are represented, or when different categories of impairment are sampled, both of which might result in two or more stable sequences which occur, however, in a different order (Williams *et al.* 1976). A non-cumulative dimension, on the other hand, would be one in which a number of indices worsen simultaneously.

Where, however, a single stable sequence or cumulative scale is found in disability, it has advantages as a health indicator. The first advantage is in the non-arbitrary rank ordering which is deducible for conforming cases. This deduction rests on the explanation of the evidence in terms of a progressive cumulative loss of activities (so that an individual only adds a new disability as he reaches a severer stage), and in terms of the similarity and predictability of the progression across conforming individuals (so that the nature and severity of each stage is common to all of them). Note that this explanation of the evidence, from which the rank order can be deduced, is not necessarily the only one possible; but it is a simple and plausible explanation which has no immediate competitors as yet.

A second advantage of detecting cumulative sequences lies in the fact that the interesting cases who do not conform can be identified, and the reasons for their non-conformity investigated. This faculty of identifying its own errors is an important virtue of the method, especially where individual justice is an important consideration.

The chief disadvantage of the method is the fact that its product is not an interval scale but a rank order. But in an area of measurement which has often suffered from excessively arbitrary assumptions, modesty may be the best policy.

PROGRESS IN CUMULATIVE SCALING 1973–79

The germ of the theoretical idea that disability cumulates goes back to work done by Katz and others (1963). However, Katz did not cast the patterns he observed in a strictly cumulative form, and the earliest use of cumulative scaling for disability seems to have been made by Skinner and Yett (1973) not on any particular theoretical hypothesis but as a method of minimising the number of disability categories in their analysis. Katz's hypothesis was finally tested by cumulative scaling in 1976 on data from Lambeth (Williams *et al.* 1976), and it was confirmed.

Next year Bebbington (1977) confirmed the existence of cumulative scales in measurements of the disabled population of Kensington and Chelsea, and a year later Barlow and Matthews (1978) confirmed that they existed in personal tasks performed by the elderly respondents of the OPCS national survey reported by Hunt in 1978. Barlow and Matthews also confirmed a scale in women's domestic tasks, but not in men's. At the same time Cairns (1977, 1978) and Williams (1979) confirmed scales in the national surveys conducted by the Institute of Social and Economic Research at York. In this last case the Lambeth scales were replicated as part of the work. Finally, work is currently in hand to replicate the Lambeth scales in the Harris national survey of 1968–9.

This is all progress, though as one might expect from the dates of each contribution it is progress on large-scale survey data already in existence and collected on earlier models of item relevance. It has been noted that for the purposes of survey assessment of disabled populations the earlier rule-of-thumb methods do not differ much from each other or from the results of cumulative scaling (Williams *et al.* 1976, Bebbington 1977).

By contrast, the specific improvements hoped for in the development of cumulative scaling as a health indicator were in the comparison of groups or individuals for whom alternative benefits, services, treatments or disposals were contemplated, or whose changes over time were an important feature. In these respects the results from the York study of institutional and home care for the elderly, now nearing completion, should be important. Similarly data have been collected on alternative hospital regimes, from which some early results were published in Williams *et al.* (1976), but so far samples have been very small, and constitute only a very small beginning in clinical uses of the scaling. Changes over time, likewise, were obtainable on a small part of the York data, and the temporal aspect ought to receive more extensive treatment in the future.

This, in brief, is how far cumulative scaling has developed in terms of the objectives originally envisaged. There are, however, problems as well and these are not merely technical but also conceptual, and cast light on what is presupposed in the use of a scaling method. The remainder of what I say will be devoted to these problems, first stating five apparently local technical difficulties, then drawing out the theoretical implications, and in conclusion, relating these implications to other theories of valuation.

PROBLEMS IN THE DEVELOPMENT STILL TO BE OVERCOME

The first limitation of what has been done is that items have some-times had a *logical* relationship built into them. The 1976 scale was not free from this limitation as the bedfast item had by logical necessity to rank below the other mobility items. Similarly in Bebbington's items the category 'can with difficulty' *logically* preceded 'cannot'. Of course, having some logical relationships between items does not ensure that all items fall under one concept, but it helps — and the more help is gained from such items the more the confirmation of one concept approximates a truism which is therefore of little interest.

Secondly there has been a great variety of items used, and there is a danger in this of capitalising on chance conformities to a scaling pattern. At the extreme this can give rise to the belief that *any* set of disability items ought to scale, and there have been one or two disillusionments because of this. Disillusion for this reason is in-appropriate, because there must be some theoretical expectation that we are dealing with one concept. But perhaps more dangerous is successful scaling of items which have no good reason to scale. If this is the result of chance on a one-off collection of items, it will delay the process of establishing what sequences of disability are stable and in what conditions. An important place must therefore be given to replication.

Thirdly, obtaining a scale is not a conclusive demonstration that there is one concept present, even when the interference of chance is excluded. It is a little like the problem of factor analysis — too often a factor can be found for items which do not seem to have a conceptual expression. Scaling is the tool of a conceptual hypothesis, not its origin. In disability the important conceptual distinctions already current have been between types of diagnostic or symptom-atic conditions, types of impairment and limb function, and types of activity described in terms of the ends of daily life. It is only the last of these that can be assigned ranks of handicap. The first two classifications are essentially causal concepts. There may be a case for mixing items from these three classifications in a standard ADL test, as is often done, but in scaling only one classification should be used, and in scaling to assess handicap only the last classification should be used. There is still a tendency to blur these concepts – for instance, in Williams *et al.* (1976) 'limb function' mobility items such as sitting and standing were used as proxies for a range of ends of daily living.

Fourthly, the activities so far studied are not in any sense complete as a conception of daily living. New items, especially the capacity to communicate, need to be included. As well as replication, a process of gradual expansion of items is required. At some point, however, the limits of the cumulative phenomenon will emerge and some items which are undoubtedly 'disability' items will prove to belong to a different kind of phenomenon. Such a finding will be theoretically informative, and will make it necessary to elucidate the concepts involved more carefully.

Finally, there arise situations in which we are confident before scaling that we have one concept, and we are more interested in the extent to which that concept is cumulative. Barlow and Matthews distinguished homogeneous sex roles, and the domestic items appropriate to each of them, by an alternative statistical analysis. They therefore felt justified in asking simply how cumulative the men's items were, taking it as proven that they fell under a single concept. Obtaining only a 'quasi-scale' as it is termed, that is only a moderate ordering, they nevertheless used this as a basis for ranking since they were concerned only with general results. But when is this legitimate and when not?

These five problems cannot be resolved without raising again the crucial importance of the theoretical assumptions which lead us to expect a single cumulative phenomenon.

THE NEED FOR THEORETICAL EXPLICITNESS IN RESOLVING THE PROBLEMS

It has been suggested that three causal models underlie current work on disability, and two of these could lead to the logical requirement of cumulation (Williams 1979). One is implicit in Barlow & Matthews (1978 pp. 6–7) where 'necessary physical movement' is seen as cumulative: 'tasks requiring bending and stretching (cause) most difficulty, and those requiring detailed manipulation the least'. They do not test this proposition, however, and attempts to define and test a cumulative order of mechanical impairment have not so far proved very successful as explanations of cumulation in disabilities of daily living.

The second model proposes that the deviant position of the disabled is 'normalised' by offering them a temporary social identity on a curriculum of recovery. This, like the learning curriculum by which children are socialised, is cumulative. Cumulation, therefore, is socially produced, and it occurs in activities which are obligatory for adults to perform by themselves. There is some support for this model.

On either of these models, though, cumulative scaling is not just a logical convenience applicable to putting order into any set of data on disability. It is the discovery of a stable and replicable order 'out there' which incidentally permits us to make many necessary judgements of handicap. Either a concept of impairment is involved, which is an attempt to describe *natural* phenomena, and is subject to correction by those phenomena; or a concept of handicap is involved, which is an attempt to describe *social* phenomena, and is subject to correction by those phenomena in the same way.

These conceptual hypotheses and empirical corrections will make it possible to define the extent of the cumulative phenomenon in disability more accurately. In exploring the extent of it, two opposite procedures may be relevant, though we cannot usually employ both satisfactorily on the same items of the same data. The first is relevant when there is good reason to think that an item *may* be a member of a cumulative concept, but insufficient reason to say that it must be. An example, using the deviance model, is incontinence. Continence is an obligatory social accomplishment, but there is some doubt whether it is defined as a voluntary action, and therefore re-learnable in the same way as dressing. If incontinence scales with other obligatory and voluntary activities, that is evidence for its inclusion. Quasi-scales are unacceptable here.

The second procedure is relevant when there is good reason to say that an item *must* be a member of a cumulative concept. The evidence will usually include the fact that it has been found to scale in a more general context than the one considered. An example might be that obligatory domestic tasks have been found to scale, but the behaviour of those living alone is found to vary. In this case the interest lies in how far the cumulative curriculum is successfully imposed by informal social pressures, and quasi-scales and even absence of scaling are topics in themselves, not merely failed scales.

CONCLUSION

This assessment of cumulative scaling raises a final question about the theoretical relationships of the principal scaling approaches. Broadly, in the psychometric approaches the assumption must be taken that the judgement made in abstraction to rules chosen by the researcher is the same as the judgement which would be made in the various actual contexts in which a health state is experienced. The imposition of what the researcher regards as the appropriate rules of choice is particularly clear in this case, and it is an important source of doubt about the method's validity.

'Revealed preference' is a way of getting round this problem — surely by looking at the way people behave when they are given alternatives, and seeing which alternatives they choose, one can arrive at a sound statement of their preferences? The answer is not as simple as it seems. If the people concerned are engaged in evaluating and choosing freely between the alternatives perceived by the researcher, then of course he can say something about their preferences; but if they do not perceive some of the alternatives or act automatically without any previous evaluation of the alternatives, it is hard to see how preferences can be invoked as an explanation. Most tantalising of all, perhaps, is a situation somewhere between these two possibilities, when a degree of pressure or coercion is brought to bear on the actor. It is valid in one sense of the word 'preference' to explain the actor's decision in this case as his preference — but is that the sense in which policy makers wish to know about the preferences of their client? A method of weighting health states by revealed preference must surely invoke the policy maker's sense; but that, as with psychometric scaling, though in a slightly different sense, presupposes that the researcher's rules of choice are being followed. Inconsistent use of those rules can of course be identified, but that is not the point. Behaviour consistent with the rules but at odds with 'real' preferences in the policy maker's sense is all too possible. With both the psychometric approach and with revealed preference, a hazardous assumption about preferences is made which is not empirically tested.

By analogy, the basis of cumulative scaling might be described as a 'revealed norm', an assumption that an area of behaviour is governed by a single cumulative concept; but by contrast that assumption is a hypothesis which is put to an empirical test. The confirmation of the scaling hypothesis in disability since 1976 is encouraging in this respect. But how far is the rank ordering thus achieved able to tell the policy-maker what he wants to know about 'real' preferences? A norm in sociology is frankly admitted to being anything from a uniformity of behaviour based on free preferences to one which is the result of punitive corporate pressures. The precise kind of norm involved is very important in the field of disability as in any situation where some people are relatively powerless — should we use valuations of health states which reflect the priorities of disabled people as individuals or those which reflect the rules of priority which they negotiate with the people round them? To answer such questions in the 'revealed norm' approach, tools of analysis are needed which can separate the very complex meanings of preferences within normal behaviour in natural settings.

It seems therefore that each of the three major approaches may have a similar problem of identifying 'real' preferences. In exploring this problem, my own inclination is naturally to start from the area in which steady findings do appear to be possible, that is, from the 'revealed norms' of people's behaviour in defining and organising handicap. Whether, when and in what sense these norms can be said to represent revealed preferences must then be stated as the initial problem. Included in that problem are at least the following questions.

(1) To what extent do the actors in this context act automatically on a received 'recipe'?
(2) What otherwise are the actors' definitions of alternative courses open to them?
(3) To what extent do they accept an authority in making their choices, and how far is that acceptance a preference?
(4) What further constraints are placed upon them by others' preferences, and do these constitute 'unfair' constraints?

The exploration of these questions may, and probably will, be illuminated in turn by the posing of hypothetical questions such as those in which ingenious applications of economic theory and psychophysics have already been made. But it seems to me that so far we know too little about the assumed and actual contexts to which these hypothetical questions are relevant, and that more theoretical knowledge of behaviour in actual contexts might help to define whose preferences are expressed in what norms. To reflect popular norms correctly, simply and without arbitrariness is one valid attribute of a health indicator, and this the cumulative scaling of disability can achieve; but to reflect how norms bear on individual preferences is a subtler and more radical task, and to further it we may now need to look much closer at the groups and networks surrounding disabled people and the way they work in their natural settings.

11

Socio-Political Issues in the Use of Health Indicators

DONALD PATRICK and SALLY GUTTMACHER

Interest in the development and use of social indicators for health policy decisions in developed countries has arisen from four major historical trends. The first, and perhaps most important, has been the shifting nature and distribution of disease and death. In many parts of the third world, extremely low standards of living are associated with higher rates of infectious disease and lower life expectancy. In the more developed, industrialized nations, however, there has been a considerable decline in overall mortality from infectious disease and a concomitant rise in disability due to chronic illness. This changing pattern has been attributed to the pervasive influence of social and economic factors on disease prevalence such as better nutrition, housing, immunization, and public health hygiene and sanitation (McKeown 1980). As these products of economic development bring a decline in mortality and an increase in life expectancy, the population balance has tipped toward the elderly.

The importance of this trend for indicator development is tied to the changing role of medicine and the growing efforts of the health care system to prolong the life of people with *non-avoidable* illness. An increasing range of caring services is being directed toward persons with arthritis, back pain, respiratory ailments, and other chronic conditions. One result of this expansion is the search for indicators that will reflect the output or value of these caring services.

The emphasis on caring services is reflected in the abundance of indicators based on the operationalized measures of one's ability to carry out usual activities, reports of acute illness and injury, and medically diagnosed chronic conditions. The majority of proposed health indicators have been concerned with negative health, that is the impact of disease or impairment and intervention on the functioning of an individual or the population. Indicators of 'positive' health or those behaviours or conditions which actually promote a higher level of well-being have been difficult to develop or apply. Elinson (1980) has also noted that indicators of non-manifest disease, preclinical or clinical, which is free of symptoms and not yet interfering with social functioning (such as neoplasms, diabetes, and hypertension), have been neglected. Without such indicators, disease prevention, particularly of asymptomatic chronic disease which is potentially disabling or fatal, will not be possible. The policy emphasis on evaluating the effectiveness of caring services, therefore, has determined the direction of indicator development with the possible consequences of limiting change in social policy.

A second historical trend is the increasing size and complexity of modern health services. Health care systems, whether government-sponsored, private or pluralistic, involve mammoth organizations with multiple administrative tiers and a complex set of activities. Increasing complexity has spurred the search for answers to how services can be better organized and conducted. The continued growth of medical services and technology, such as computed tomographic (CAT) scanning and therapeutic methodologies such as coronary bypass surgery, renal dialysis and heart transplantation have led decision-makers and the public to ask questions about the appropriateness, effectiveness and limits of new technologies. Indicators of effectiveness are desired to address the questions involved in using the new technologies for various ends.

The third major historical trend motivating the policy use of health indicators is increasing expenditure on health services. In most Western nations, the proportion of the GNP spent on health care has risen over the last decade. In the United Kingdom, public and private, capital and current health care expenditure consumed 3.9 per cent of the GNP in 1950 and 5.5 in 1975. In the United States, these figures were 4.5 in 1950 and 8.6 in 1975 (Maxwell 1981).

From early in this century, national discussions have taken place in the United States on the economic implications of illness. Fisher (1909) estimated the annual losses to the economy from morbidity and mortality that he hypothesized could be reduced through preventive medicine and better hygiene and sanitation. Fisher's work illustrated the need for increased public investment in health services, and influenced others to determine the 'money value of a man' (Dublin and Lotka 1930).

As health care expenditures have risen, most notably in the United States, cost containment has become the 'war cry' of the policy maker, the administrator and sometimes clinicians themselves. Politicians from all political parties believe that it is no longer feasible to continue pumping a greater proportion of resources into the health care system without increased accountability. Indicators are being proposed to cut costs in areas where treatment is apparently less effective and to assess the economic burden that might result from no treatment at all. Thus, health indicators could be used to support the contention that if services are cut in the public or private sector to control cost, the health status of the population may not be affected. In some cases, this may be correct. Were services such as unnecessary surgery to be reduced, health status might improve (Bunker *et al.* 1977). In other instances, any ineffectiveness reflected in health status indicators might be due to the lack of access to health services. For example, a recent analysis in the United States suggests that 'there has been a narrowing of the gap between the poor and non-poor in the utilization of health services during the same period that there has been a widening of the gap in health status' (Wilson and White 1977).

The last major historical trend motivating the use of indicators is the vast expansion of government in health policy over the past century. The move toward more regulated policy and planning from the 'top down' is predicated on a conception of social justice and the assurance that each person in society receives a fair and equal share of both the burdens and benefits of that society (Beauchamp 1976). The question should be: what set of principles might be used in dividing the burdens and benefits and finding a consensus on what is fair and equal? Policy-makers are requesting indicators to provide criteria for allocating burdens and benefits on a national, area or local basis. Standards in respect to the appropriate supply, distribution and organization of health resources are expressions of health goals in quantitative terms. Health status measures are required for resource allocation, certification-of-need, equal access, and quality-cost assessment.

These historical trends, then — the increasing burden of chronic illness, the growing complexity of health care services and technology, rapidly rising health care expenditure, and the move toward an expanded role of government in policy and service provision — have motivated the development of indicators. But what assumptions do these proposed indicators make and what might be some of the social and political implications for their use when examined against this brief historical background?

IMPLICATIONS AND ASSUMPTIONS

State-of-health indicators explicitly or implicitly operationalize prevailing definitions of health. And definitions of health, at any time, are likely to reflect the ideology and culture of the most powerful groups in society. As noted earlier, many definitions of health have centred on *productive functioning* whether it be 'capacity of an individual for the effective performance of the roles and tasks for which he has been socialized' (Parsons, 1972) or the more recent attempts to move from fitness and capacity to performance and behaviour (Patrick *et al.* 1973). The norm from which deviation is noted is the productive role of wage labour, school, leisure or housework. Bed-disability, restricted activity or work-lost days are examples of routinely available indicators based on such functional definitions. Although these functional definitions imply activities other than wage-earning, the notion of maintenance of health as investment is closely tied to capacity or ability (Grossman 1972).

One major reason for the focus on 'productivity' definitions is acceptance of a traditional medical model, both in terms of the aetiology of disease and the 'engineering' approach toward care of the body. Operational measures of health status concentrate on the impact on function after the individual has been affected by disease or impairment. Limiting definitions to the mechanisms of disease rather than to the circumstances of its genesis is also tied to a reliance on the development of technology in medical care. Lewis Thomas (1975) calls this 'half-way technology': doing things after the fact may prolong life for a few years but will not alter the cause of disease.

The curative perspective may also deflect attention away from a critical appraisal of those aspects of society such as tobacco and alcohol advertising, industrial waste and pollution, and job hazards and stress that have been directly or indirectly linked to a increased risk of disease and death. At best, when data are aggregated, the impact of possible stressors on function can be examined; at worst, by focusing on individual well-being, there is a danger that the individual will be blamed for selecting a particular life style or course of action and thereby determining his or her own state of health. For example, early data on the effectiveness of ante-natal care indicated that many women did not attend clinics or classes and that low attendance was associated with poor pregnancy outcome. The initial reaction of providers was to blame the mothers for what was described as stupid and irresponsible behaviour (McKinlay and McKinlay 1972).

Another major implication of using social indicators for planning is the question of privacy and access to the information on which indicators are based. The ethical problems of collecting health data for planning and evaluation are increasingly being discussed (Home Office 1978). It is important to recognize that privacy may not be equally distributed across all the classes in our society and the cloak of privacy may benefit the privileged as against the under-privileged. As Douglas (1968) notes in relation to official statistics on suicide, the power to control public access to and classification of private events rises with social status, perhaps throwing a significant skew into official statistics.

Perhaps the major assumption and implication of using state-of-health indicators for planning lies in the logic of forging policy directions on the basis of indicators. Indicators can never substitute for the political process of deciding what to do now about inequalities between groups, about the participation of different groups in decision-making, or about the priorities of action. Nor should efforts to protect the health of the general public be deflected or retarded by the *lack* of health status measures. Answers to questions such as 'What level of health is acceptable to the public?' cannot be determined by scientific means. Policy decisions, whatever the data to support them, are the product of broad social conditions, struggles and influences of society. As McKeown (1980) has written recently:

So long as the deleterious influences are not eliminated, either because they are unrecognized, as in breast cancer, or because we are unable or unwilling to accept their removal, as in the case of road accidents, there will be need for continued treatment of diseases and disabilities which in principle are *avoidable*. Indeed, some of the greatest successes of clinical medicine are in treatment of conditions such as accidents which, ideally, should not occur.

TOWARD OPTIMUM HEALTH INDICATORS

The major question given the motivation for indicators and their assumptions and implications is how to safeguard against any potential or actual pernicious effects of using indicators for policy decisions that may not be in the public interest. First of all, it should be recognized that the development of statistical tools for health planning is not an end in itself: it is only the means for promoting the health and quality of life of all members of society. Improvement of a data base, research instrument or planning tool should be viewed in this light. Although such a statement might seem self-evident, funding agents, researchers and data analysts have sometimes been too concerned with developing new techniques to gain a slightly better measure of what seems already clear.

For example, traditional indicators, such as infant mortality statistics, tell a great deal about variations in the distribution of health and disease promoting conditions. Such statistics indicate that there are dramatic differences in the prospects for children according to their socio-economic position and ethnic status. Children born in lower class families are at greater risk from birth. Morbidity data tell the same story, even though they may be somewhat less reliable than mortality statistics. Persons living in conditions of poverty are less healthy and less apt to remain well. The major cause of such disparity can be traced to class differences in living conditions, in access to care, and in some cases to use of services. Problems of measurement should not detract from the use of all such information to correct maldistribution of services and resources and disparities in the health status of poor persons.

It is also important that health indicators measure at least some of those aspects of health that programmes and policies can affect. The development of more sensitive assessments of cognitive function or development, for instance, may simply be academic exercises unless such measures are tested on programmes instituted and sustained to achieve positive impact upon such function. Health indicators that are sensitive to intervention are notoriously difficult to construct and interpret, since the provision of health care and factors outside the health sector can adversely influence traditional measures of health (Martini *et al.* 1979). Nevertheless, the promise of indicators cannot be realized without actual tests of policies and programmes.

To avoid misplaced precision and improve the usefulness of indicators more systematic attention might be given to the process of indicator development itself. Scientists, politicians, philosophers, health professionals, consumers and bureaucrats all have an interest in health indicators. The objectives of indicator development, however, are not always agreed by the developers and users. Both historical and policy-analytic studies of the 'who and why' of health indicators might provide a sociology of science which could in turn improve and hasten indicator development.

Secondly, to safeguard the public interest, health indicators should be tied to a conception of social process and social structure that is specified within a clearly identified value system. The importance of hypothesizing the relationships which may exist between social structure, social process and state-of-health is illustrated by recent work on the effect of unemployment on health. Brenner (1977, 1979) has analyzed the variation in annual overall mortality rates for the USA, England, Wales and Sweden in relation to changes in the annual level of unemployment. He argues that unemployment, with a five-year lag, impacts on health by firstly reducing family income and material standard of living and secondly by reducing people's sense of meaning and purpose at work and making them more vulnerable to ill health. Eyer (1977) has challenged this analysis by arguing that the health impact of unemployment is much shorter than the five-year lag allowed by Brenner. On the contrary, Eyer argues that death rates increase when business booms and employment is high because economic booms induce worker migration, weaken social ties, increase stress and increase alcohol and tobacco consumption. Eyer further argues that social networks are strong when the economy is depressed, thus protecting people's health. These two analysts clearly have different conceptions of social structure and social process that have permitted competing interpretations of covariation in economic and mortality indicators. The results from these studies therefore must be assessed both in the context of the social system model used by the investigators and that of the possible ambiguity of existing data bases for testing hypotheses about what is causing what (and through what mechanism).

A promising development in the publication and analysis of health indicators within a socio economic context is the *Prevention Profile* (Department of Health and Human Services 1980) which presents the successes, failures and gaps in health promotion and disease prevention in the United States during the recent past. The report shows that the benefits of prevention have reached different groups of the US population unevenly, such as excessive deaths from homicide in young non-white males and the rising death rate among women from cancers of the respiratory system related to the increase in women smokers. In the United Kingdom, *Inequalities in Health* (Department of Health and Social Security 1980) shows that health inequalities have not diminished and, in some cases, they may be increasing since the inception of the National Health Service. The presentation of data for different social classes, age groups, geographical areas and other socio-economic characteristics helped to pinpoint those groups for whom the pace of reducing already identified risk factors must be accelerated.

A third means of safeguarding the public interest concerns the incorporation of values in the indicators or indexes. The choice of a conception of health, the selection of dimensions, the construction of an indicator or index, and the proposed use of the indicator all imply problems of valuation that are unavoidable. As a number of philosophers of science have recognized (including Kaplan 1964, p. 387) values cannot be excluded from science, and the 'problem for methodology is not *whether* values are involved in inquiry, but *which*, and above all, *how* they are to be empirically grounded'.

Any indicator or index applied to populations for determining health status or to health programmes for evaluating outcomes must confront the question of *who* prefers *which* states of health under *which* circumstances? A composite profile or index requires the aggregation of multiple individual descriptors into summary scores. Researches may impose their own value weighting system upon combinations of descriptors, use data analytic techniques to score the descriptors according to their frequency of occurrence, or obtain weights for the descriptors in scaling studies using utility models, psychometrics, or empirical social decision valuation (Patrick 1979). A socio-medical health metric that fairly represents society's preferences will be necessary to move indicators from methodological testing to application in programme evaluation, priority setting and resource allocation.

Fair and democratic representation of society's value or preference for states of health requires that samples of community values be obtained. Preference judgements attached to conditions of life have most often been pre-empted by physicians and other health professionals. The use of physicians as judges has been justified on the grounds that physicians have a better understanding of the nature of health conditions than lay persons and moreover that the medical value system is one that has been imputed to society (Raiffa 1968). Some decisions require professional judgement, such as the estimation of prognoses. Strong empirical evidence is required, however, before accepting that the values of physicians or other professionals represent the community. Additional effort is required to measure consumer opinion and decisions about personal health and health care. Such work would make it possible to compare provider and customer preferences and values of different social groups and communities.

Lastly, changing definitions of health and illness would follow from a public health ethic more strongly based on principles of social justice recognizing that only by collective action can those aspects of social organisation that are damaging to health be changed. Effort is needed to relate social definitions of health to participation in social or community life. Such indicators might be more sociological in that clinical categories would be combined with the individual's social situation as well as functioning. Assessments of health might then be combined with other indicators of social and economic conditions so that disability or dysfunction can be assessed in terms of handicap or disadvantage (World Health Organization 1980).

The translation of concepts into indicators will take place within the ideological and political context of the researcher and decision-maker. Those of us working in the field of health indicator development will need to recognize, assess and incorporate explicit socio-political issues into our work if health is to be defined and measured on a different set of assumptions.

12

Implicit Values in Administrative Decisions[1]

J W HURST and G H MOONEY

INTRODUCTION

This paper argues that health status measurement is value laden, that currently, although not necessarily explicitly, weights are being placed on different states-of-health by the *producers* of health care and that *their* 'demand functions' can be utilized in devising a scaling system of health status measurement. Through the 'revealed preferences' of the administrative decision-making process, much can be learned about these producers' demand functions but little empirical research has yet been done on this approach to weighting of health status. Consequently this paper is largely exploratory in nature.

DEMAND, NEED, AND THE WEIGHTING OF STATES-OF-HEALTH

One of the major difficulties with health status measurement is that it is not value free. Different systems of health care delivery have different objectives and priorities. Before it is possible to begin generally to get to grips with health status measurement *per se* it is necessary to answer such questions as: what are the objectives in providing care for the elderly? What weight should be given to care of the elderly vis-à-vis care of other client groups, and to different sub-objectives within this client group? How are the dimensions of these objectives and sub-objectives to be considered?

But if health status measurement is not value-free, nor in turn the

---

1. © Crown Copyright

answering of these types of questions, then whose values are to be assumed to be most relevant in such valuation? Traditionally economists have tended to the view that the individual consumer's preferences should reign – the concept of 'consumer sovereignty'. Mishan (1972), for example, suggests that 'economists are generally agreed – either as a canon of faith, as a political tenet, or as an act of expediency – to accept the dictum that each person knows his own interest best'.

It is on the basis of this view that the economists' concept of demand (that is willingness to pay on the part of a consumer) has been constructed with its underlying concept of 'utility' or satisfaction. The more 'utility' an individual expects to obtain from a particular good or service the more he will be willing to pay for it. Unfortunately, and not unexpectedly (since 'utility' has occasionally been equated with happiness), there are very considerable problems involved in measuring utility. Nonetheless the concept has been found to be very useful in economics and indeed it has been suggested (through the theory of revealed preference) that by studying individuals' behaviour with regard to changing prices and/or incomes it may be possible to measure utility, since such behaviour reveals individuals' relative preferences for different packages of goods and services.

Indeed, the use of utility theory in health status measurement has been advocated by others, notably Torrance (1976b). He has, for example, attempted to explore 'the extent to which utility theory can provide a theoretical foundation for health status index models', arguing that if such a foundation can be developed it would be useful in a number of ways including 'how to establish the weights for health states'. However, Torrance appears not to have developed it in the particular direction advocated in this paper.

However far we might be prepared to go in accepting the concept of consumer sovereignty in respect of some goods and services, it is unlikely, in the context of the good 'health', that we would be prepared to go all the way.

One possible reason for questioning the role of consumer sovereignty is the existence of the so-called 'agency relationship' whereby patients delegate decisions about their treatment to doctors. However, in a 'pure' agency relationship the doctor supplies only technical skills in advising and treating the patient. All the values and preferences affecting the treatment come from the patient. There are reasons to believe that, in practice, the communication of patients' preferences to doctors is quite imperfect. One study, for example, suggested that doctors, in recommending treatment for lung cancer, took insufficient account of patients' attitudes to risk (McNeil *et al.* 1978). There are also reasons for suspecting that, in many circumstances, doctors' financial interests, or their own preferences, affect treatment (Tuoy and Wolfson 1977). The pervasiveness of such departures from the pure agency relationship is difficult to judge. Nonetheless, in a well regulated medical profession it should be possible, in principle, for the agency relationship to complement rather than conflict with consumer sovereignty.

What is more problematic (for consumer sovereignty) is that in most societies governments have stepped in first with programmes to provide health care to those least able to care for themselves, such as the poor and mentally ill, and then with programmes to provide equitable access to health services by whole populations. Such programmes seldom rely on cash transfers. Rather, they provide 'free' access to services in kind or subsidised health insurance, both of which offer consumers relatively unconstrained access to a wide range of health services. In either case there tends to be excess demand for services and various forms of non-price rationing take the place of the market. Paternalism tends to supplant consumer sovereignty and the argument moves further away from the concept of demand, based on consumer preferences, to that of need, or merit, based on social or providers' preferences.

But why with health should there be this element of intervention/ interference with consumer sovereignty? Why should the concept of demand be less appropriate in health care than elsewhere in the economy? There are a number of reasons for this. Partly these stem from the view that the good 'health' is subject to such uncertainty and irrationality that individual consumers are unable (indeed may be unwilling) to exercise appropriate preferences themselves; partly it is because of the existence of 'externalities': not only those associated with immunisation procedures but also 'humanitarian externalities' (that is as Culyer (1976) puts it, 'Individuals are affected by others' health status for the simple reason that *most of them care*'); and partly, continuing with the distributional aspect just introduced by the mention of externalities, because of the view that individuals ought to have a right to health care.

The move from the concept of demand to that of need potentially raises enormous problems because this latter concept appears to have been defined in as many ways as there are individuals who have examined it. (See, for example, Williams 1978.) However, and it is all that matters in the context of this paper, a common denominator in all such definitions is the involvement of providers (for example the medical profession, politicians and administrators). It can be argued, for example, that in many · health care systems the main influence on defining need comes from within the health care system itself and that consequently the *values* underlying need (and hence health status) are drawn from this source.

The introduction of the concept of need does not so much invalidate the concept of demand but rather emphasizes that the relevant 'actor' in the demand function is not the consumer but the provider or decision makers in the health care system 'acting' on behalf of the consumer. In turn this means that in determining the ideal output of different health care services we are ultimately interested in the demand (the willingness to pay) of the provider for different states-of-health for the (eventual) consumers. This would then provide us with what Culyer, Lavers and Williams (1971) have called 'the calculation of an *intensity of need* measure which states the intensity with which "Society" needs each of a variety of states-of-health'.

There are essentially two aspects to health status measurement: the description of states-of-health and the scaling or weighting. This paper is concerned with the latter — taking as its basis that the revealed preferences from within the health care system can indicate the existing, albeit often non-explicit, weights placed on different states-of-health. In doing so it recognises the major role carved out for the public sector in the financing and provision of health care in so many countries.

REVEALED PREFERENCE AND IMPLICIT WEIGHTS

Writing more than 30 years ago, Samuelson (1948) suggested that:

> the economic theory of consumer's behaviour can be largely built up on the notion of 'revealed preference'. By comparing the costs of different combinations of goods at different relative price situations, we can infer whether a given batch of goods is preferred to another batch; the individual guinea-pig, by his market behaviour, reveals his preference patterns — if there is such a consistent pattern.

This proposition stimulated a fairly vigorous debate in the economic journals and, nearly 30 years later, McFadden (1975) attempted to apply this originally consumer oriented concept to the revealed preferences of a government bureaucracy. He writes:

> Government bureaucracies responsible for regulating utilities or designing investment projects are often given the general mandate to maximize 'public welfare' and left with considerable freedom in translating this goal into concrete decision rules. The result is often an ambiguity within the organisation about the weight to be given to various factors in making choices, leading to decisions which are vulnerable to criticism on grounds of inconsistency or lack of fidelity to the mandate.

McFadden suggests two ways of assessing organizational performance of a bureaucracy: first the study of the *process* of decision-making and secondly to approach such assessment from the point of view of examining 'the *consequence* or *outcomes* of the organization's decisions, and to pose the *revealed preference* question of whether there exists an implicit choice criterion such that the bureaucracy behaves *as if* it is attempting to follow this choice rule'.

Now in the context of health care there is frequently the notion of the health service attempting to 'maximize "public welfare"', that is in this context attempting to maximize health (or perhaps more accurately the utility or satisfaction from health care outputs). Again, the idea embraced in McFadden's second approach to assessing the performance of an organization of examining 'outcomes' has its parallel in health care of examining the 'health outcomes' to see whether there is an implicit choice criterion underlying these. This leads directly into the issue of health status measurement in that an examination of such a criterion can provide an indication of the *weights* being attached, at least implicitly, to particular types of states of health.

Put more simply if it can be shown that, in equilibrium, the cost of a unit of health output a is twice that of the cost of a unit of health output b, then, by implication, the underlying choice criterion is such that the weight being attached to the latter output is half that of the former. We then have a mechanism for adding together different types of health output, for example lives extended by renal dialysis and the care of elderly people in residential homes.

More accurately, we need to deal with costs *at the margin* (that is of some variation in the output produced). For example, if a screening programme is selective, in the sense of screening high risk cases first and then progressively lower risk cases, the implied value of detecting a diseased case will increase as lower and lower risk groups are screened. Given a decision to screen risk group i but not to extend it to risk group j (where the former have a slightly higher risk than the latter) the decision has been made implicitly to expend £x per diseased case detected but not £y (where $y > x$). In this example, the value being attached to detecting a diseased case is at least £x but something less than £y. Thus an examination *ex post* of bureaucratic decision-making, relating costs to output *at the margin* of different programmes, will allow a system of weighting to be derived. (Similarly, a presentation of such data *ex ante* will force on decision-makers an explicit recognition of the relative weights involved in deciding upon which risk groups to screen).

Clearly, it is unlikely in the *ex post* situation that it will be discovered that for like outputs the marginal costs will always be the same. Rather in such circumstances we would anticipate that such marginal costs will be distributed about some mean or 'location'. As McFadden suggests: 'The "location" of this distribution provides information on the average weighting of factors in decisions, while its "dispersion" gives a measure of the internal consistency of the bureaucracy's decision structure.'

If such 'locations' can be identified they can then be used as weights for different health outcomes – *given* an acceptance that the health care system is genuinely attempting to maximize welfare with the resources at its disposal. At the same time if the 'dispersions' can be identified there is scope for improving the *efficiency* of health care programmes.

To pursue the 'locations' issue in more detail, let us examine the following hypothetical and much simplified example. Let us assume that there are only two types of health output, a and b, which are provided by health care programmes A and B respectively and that the costs of such provision are as shown in table 12.1.

Now let us further assume that under the existing decision-making process five units of output a are being produced and five units of output b, giving a total expenditure to the two programmes of £1600 (that is £500 to A and £1100 to B) and that this is the preferred combination. Now by implication we have here the 'revealed preference' of the bureaucracy for a as compared with b. *At the margin* the cost of a unit of a is £100 and of b £200, a ratio of *1:2*. This implies that a unit of b is weighted approximately twice as highly as a unit of a – since it would be possible to reduce the output of programme B by *one* unit and expand the output of programme A by *two* units within the *same* total expenditure. Obviously

TABLE 12.1 *Cost of health care programmes*

Programme A			Programme B		
Units of output a	Total cost £	Marginal cost £	Units of output b	Total cost £	Marginal cost £
1	100	100	1	300	300
2	200	100	2	550	250
3	300	100	3	750	200
4	400	100	4	900	150
5	500	100	5	1100	200
6	600	100	6	1350	250
7	700	100	7	1650	300
8	800	100	8	2000	350
9	900	100	9	2400	400
10	1000	100	10	2850	450

other combinations of programmes *A* and *B* are possible within the budget constraint *but* at all other possible combinations the implied ratio of *b/a* (that is the ratio of the relevant marginal costs) is either above or below two. The fact that a decision has been made to produce five of *a* and five of *b* *implies* that the weights being attached to the outputs *a* and *b* are in the ratio of approximately *1:2*. (It is of course being assumed in this example that this decision is also an 'efficient' one in the sense that values implied in this case lie on the relevant 'locations' for these types of output).

Some crude empirical examples

Comparatively little work appears to have been done on this approach to weighting different health outputs. Morley and Porter (1972) applied inverse linear programming to maternity services in Sunderland and were able to measure the implied weights attached by decision makers to various intermediate outputs. However, they did not try to measure health status itself and their work does not seem to have been developed subsequently in this direction. Most of what has been attempted has been more concerned with the issue of the 'dispersion' existing in the output 'lives saved'. In the UK for example, Mooney (1977) has shown that the implied value of life appears to vary enormously (although some of this 'dispersion' may be explicable on the basis of the non-homogeneity of the lives involved, for example children's lives as compared with adults')

Certainly much more work would be required if the approach were to become a practical tool of health status measurement.

However, a simple example can be presented for the UK of two existing policies. Buxton and West (1975) have shown that the discounted costs of providing hospital dialysis for a cohort of 1000 patients over 20 years are approximately £23 million, equivalent to a cost of approximately £3500 per year of life extended. Stilwell (1976), examining the benefits and costs of the schools' BCG vaccination programme against tuberculosis, suggests that the cost involved in preventing one case of tuberculosis is about £5500.

Both of these programmes are currently in being in the NHS. If it can be assumed (for the sake of providing an element of empiricism in this paper) that the cost figures quoted are *marginal* costs then it becomes possible to derive the relative weights implicitly attached to the outputs of these two existing programmes as in table 12.2.

TABLE 12.2 *Output/Relative Weights*

Type of output	Cost per unit of output (£)	Relative weights of output
Year of life extension for end-stage uraemia patient	3500	7
Case of TB prevented	5500	11

Or, expressing this in equivalent terms, 11 years of extended life for end-stage uraemia patients equals seven cases of TB prevented. In this way therefore an examination *ex post* of decisions on resource allocation can reveal the preference of the administrative decision-makers and allow weights to be placed on different health outputs.

It is of course possible to use information like this prospectively. For example, Hagard, Carter and Milne (1976) have indicated for the UK that if a screening programme for spina bifida cystica were introduced at a cost of about £1.2 million, it could prevent about 1,800 births of liveborn children with myelocele each year at a cost per birth of this type prevented of approximately £700. Assuming, again, that this is the marginal cost, these decision-makers in deciding whether or not to introduce such a programme would need to consider whether preventing approximately eight of such births (cost £5600) was to be weighted more highly than the prevention of one case of TB (cost £5500) or the extension of life for about 18 months for a patient with end-stage uraemia.

At a more generalized level in the NHS the *ex ante* revealed preference approach of implicit values can be seen in the use of 'norms' or 'guidelines' promulgated by the Department of Health and Social Security. These are intended to provide a framework of resource and other assumptions, and policy guidance, within which the Regional, Area and District Authorities prepare their plans. While it is possible to place different interpretations on the various aspects of these guidelines, Harris (1979) has suggested that:

> the projections of these factors – desired . . . national levels of intermediate output per head of population served, unit costs and expenditure per head of population served for various activities, and of expenditure on various commodities of groups of activities, compared to current or recent levels – have two aspects. First, they provide desired, and nationally feasible, future-year levels, which may represent central preferences (subject to national constraints) as to the relative production levels of different commodities . . . Secondly, the relative growth rates implied by the future-year figures compared to the base-year, may be intended *to signal the relative marginal benefits per £ of additional expenditure on particular activities and commodities* . . . [our italics].

Thus Harris has identified a way in which weights to be attached to particular types of outputs, or perhaps more accurately aggregations of types of outputs (such as those associated with maternity care or care of the elderly – since these are the sorts of services or programmes to which the DHSS guidelines refer) are defined *ex ante* and promulgated in a quasi-explicit fashion through these norms and guidelines.

Again, at a generalized level, the relative priority accorded to different diseases by the medical profession has already been built into the RAWP and SHARE formulae (Department of Health and Social Security, 1976, and Scottish Home and Health Department, 1977) which, for England and Scotland respectively, determine target allocations of finance to health authorities by central government. In broad terms, both formulae set out to measure, for different regions, the relative need for finance, which is based in part on the relative health status of their populations. In both formulae, part of the money for acute hospital services is shared out between health authorities in proportion (as a first approximation) to local, condition-specific crude mortality, weighted by national acute hospital bed use for each condition. In this way, the collective revealed preferences of the medical profession for treating different diseases are brought to bear, quantitatively and explicitly, on the process by which central government tries to allocate finance equitably between geographical areas.

There are thus different roles that implied values can play in health status measurement. All start from the fact that somebody or some group have made, are making, or will make, decisions on resource allocation in the health care sector that by implication involve placing weights on different health states. For decisions previously made, explicit consideration of these implied values may permit two possible courses of action. First, it may allow the decision-makers to reconsider their decisions in the light of a greater awareness of values they implied in their decisions for example to consider the question, did you really mean that a little more of output *a* was to be valued 50 times more than a little more of output *b*? Secondly, it may serve to make decision-makers more accountable in the sense of stimulating debate about whether or not the decision-makers' implied values, when made explicit, reflect those of the wider community they represent.

Again, in terms of prospective decision making, the difficulties in resource allocation in health care might be resolved more systematically if the weights implied in choosing option *A* rather than option *B* are set out explicitly so that debate can occur about what the relative weights should be for the different health outputs of the options.

At the same time, of course, it is to be hoped that the more widespread use of the approach to health status measurement would result in increased efficiency of resource allocation through a reduction in the 'dispersions' around the 'locations' (to reintroduce McFadden's terminology) of different values of health states.

FEASIBILITY OF THE APPROACH

It is worth re-emphasizing at this time that this paper is essentially about the weighting or scaling processes of health status measurement. We take the view that where certain types of public provision and finance of health services prevail it is legitimate to accept the administrative decision-making process in health care as a basis for deriving implied values and hence weights for different states-of-health. By starting from conventional utility and consumer demand theory but thereafter accepting the relevance of *producers'* demand in health care planning it is possible, in principle at least, to obtain a weighting system for health status measurement.

But how feasible is the approach? One interesting feature is that *in principle* it does not require detailed descriptions of health status per se. Since it centres on the values implicit in resource allocation decision-making, provided that there is *some* quantitative measure involved on the output side — whether it be number of tests conducted, years of life extended or even numbers of individuals affected — there is potentially fertile soil in which such analyses might be grown. However, in practice if, as a result of the implementation of the approach, decision-makers are more frequently faced with the implications of their choice on resource allocation, it is unlikely that they themselves will not demand more data regarding 'final' outputs (and indeed of consumers' preferences regarding these) and be less content with the type of 'intermediate' output data that are a common feature of current health service planning. Thus it has to be stressed that insofar as there are two main foci of health status measurement — descriptions and weighting — this paper is concerned solely with the latter.

One of the major practical difficulties in the approach outlined is that there is a plethora of levels and of individuals involved in resource allocation decision-making in any health service — and particularly in Britain. Decisions are made and influenced by central government, regional authorities, areas, districts, sectors and units; by consultative and advisory committees at national and local level; by individual clinicians; by local health councils and by the public at large. This means that there is also potentially a plethora of levels and of individuals to be studied to determine the values implied in all these different decision-making processes and levels. The nature of the choices being and to be made is also varied: choices between hospital, community and primary care services; for particular client groups such as the elderly; related to different broad objectives of health care — chronic versus acute care; on equity considerations; and about many other issues. The multi-faceted nature of such decisions and decision-making suggests that at a practical level the study of implicit values in such decisions and decision-making could be very time-consuming. However, it is potentially an advantage of the approach that it explicitly recognises the diffuse nature of decision-making on resource allocation.

Another practical difficulty is that health service decision-making takes place under uncertainty. It is not only that consumers' future health states and preferences are known imperfectly but also that decision-makers are often unsure about what the impact of any particular intervention will be on health. The effectiveness of many medical procedures is still a matter for judgement. There is evidence from one Scottish study (Hunter 1979) that under such conditions of uncertainty health service decision-makers resort to incrementalism and other rules of thumb. This may make it difficult to interview them to elicit their relative preferences for different outputs. Others have argued, in the context of patients and individuals in the population at large, that it is better to rely on the behaviour of individuals than on their feelings to assess health status (see, for example, Bergner *et al.* 1976). This may also be true of health service decision-makers.

CONCLUSION

Much of what has been said in this paper is not original, the literature on health indicators is liberally sprinkled with comments on the need to recognise the importance of values and value judgements and indeed incorporate these into health status measurement. Elsewhere, much has been written about the concept of need and its relevance to health service decision-making. However, in bringing the two together, in the context of health status measurement, we would suggest that there is value in attempting to refine and develop more comprehensively these ideas and indeed in promoting more empirical research using the approach.

13

Conclusions and Recommendations

A J CULYER

This short concluding chapter makes no attempt to summarize the foregoing. The general flavour of research in the topic of health indicators has been described in chapter one and specific aspects reviewed in considerable detail in the subsequent chapters. This chapter therefore offers some concluding comments relating to the future development of research into the topic in Europe.

The fact that this research area is very new means that, although a research programme is emerging, a clear conception of its scope will not be present in most researchers' minds so that not all potential cross-links between related parts may be identified and used. This workshop has sought to expose as many as possible of these potential linkages so as to heighten awareness.

The terminology used – and shared in common by workers from different disciplines – is not settled in its meaning and can lead to misunderstanding. Classic examples include 'health', 'indicators', 'effectiveness', 'efficiency' and 'need'. Any attempt to impose a standard usage is unlikely to meet with success. However, greater and continuing contact between European researchers would probably, in the fullness of time, lead to agreed conventions being used – or at least a clarification and better understanding of the ways researchers from different cultural and disciplinary backgrounds use their own conventions. The important thing is less to agree a common 'language' than to acquire an understanding of the various 'languages' by means of more effective communication.

The setting of research questions in the context of a general framework of the sort outlined in chapter one is probably neither explicit nor implicit in the minds of many researchers. The integrating function of such a general framework would help researchers having different specific research questions to answer, and coming from different disciplinary backgrounds, to see more clearly their own work in relation to that of others.

The multidisciplinary nature of this research field (or topic) means that the conventional lines of communication between researchers (usually set along disciplinary lines) are inadequate to support productive scholarly interchange. Instead one relies on chance contact, occasional topic-orientated (rather than the more usual discipline-oriented) conferences, and the vagaries of research contracting arrangements that may or may not throw up an evident need for joint work by people from different disciplines.

Being a 'shared' topic, health indicators research carries the inherent danger of academic 'sniping' from those seeking either to protect 'their' territory or invade that of 'others'. Neither attitude is helpful. Research sponsors — especially academic ones — should recognize that, while far from every research project will require multidisciplinary research inputs, the field is nonetheless multidisciplinary and that some problems will require explicit multidisciplinary collaboration. Among other things, this suggests that *disciplinary* based research sponsorship (for example by medical research councils) would in general *not* be a fruitful way of commissioning and responding to research proposals in this field. A single disciplinary hegemony would be utterly destructive.

Related to this is the desirability of researchers attempting to acquire acquaintanceship with the work (or the *style* of work) of researchers from other disciplines within the topic. Among other things, this implies that researchers should from time to time explicitly address colleagues in other disciplines in order to 'demystify' their own arcane art and make its methods more accessible to others. It does *not* imply we should all turn ourselves into polymaths (though if some could manage that, so much the better) but that each should have at least a lively appreciation of the modes of thought of the others.

The fact that the potential uses and users of health indicators cover broad spectra should sound an alert against attempts to narrow the focus of application arbitrarily. It implies the desirability of a *diversity* of research sponsors so that no single perception of a valid user or a unique customer can gain a hegemony. There seems, therefore, to be no case for a single *European* or individual *national* sponsoring bodies for health indicators research. A diversity of sponsors each pursuing its research interests is a healthy state of affairs, whether these be international agencies, government departments, private sponsors, or research councils.

Some work in this topic will inevitably attract no direct 'customer' prepared to act as sponsor. This is particularly true of 'pure' research in theory, method, and experimental technique. While such work can sometimes be pursued as an essential part of applied work that may have a 'customer-type' sponsor, there is a residual category of research that would normally (by analogy with discipline-specific research topics) fall to the academic research councils to sponsor. In such cases it follows that since these bodies usually have a disciplinary base (for example a *medical* research council) or group disciplines together (for example a *social science* research council) the proper procedure would be to develop within such bodies *joint* committees reflecting the varied disciplinary base of the topic.

There are a large variety of *value* issues that are not presently being addressed in the research programme – or are being addressed either in a perfunctory fashion or more seriously but by researchers who do not see themselves (and are not so seen) as being a part of the research programme. The focus on an increasing technical sophistication in indicator methodology can easily cause these issues to be lost sight of and this is probably the least satisfactory aspect of the present 'state of the art'. Here 'reform' would seem best to come from 'within'.

There is an overwhelming case for the development and sustaining of an interactive dialogue between researchers and those who may use whatever health indicators are produced (the 'customers' of research) whether they be international organizations, national governments, health policy planners and managers, or physicians in clinical practice.

From these general considerations and the more detailed discussion in the foregoing papers, two broad sets of conclusions may be drawn: one set relating to the state of scholarship in the field, the other relating to research organization.

SCHOLARSHIP

1. The scientific and informed planning of health services, as well as clinical research and practice, needs new and more sensitive indicators of 'success' or 'failure' than traditional indicators like life expectancy and infant mortality.

2. Sufficient developments already exist for health indicators or indices of a scholarly (as distinct from *ad hoc*) nature to be far more

widely incorporated into evaluative work in medical and epidemiological research (clinical trials and the like). Many who conduct
clinical trials do not avail themselves of the techniques that exist
already. Studies of the *effectiveness* of medical procedures and their
cost-effectiveness under normal operating conditions deserve, of all
health services research, the highest priority.

3. As an aid to the greater dissemination of techniques of health
measurement among medical researchers, a non-technical 'text-book'
(even 'cookbook!') would be valuable that reviewed the techniques
available and illustrated how they have been successfully employed
in the evaluation of medical procedures. Such a project from a suitably qualified author is worthy of an early claim on research funds.

4. More work is urgently needed that is directed to more macro
applications concerned, for example, with identifying priority areas
for medical research (indicators of ill-health potentially reducible by
preventive or restorative medicine but which may require medical
research before effective procedures become available) or for
resource allocation in the health services (for example identification
of client-group or regional 'needs' for resources in terms of their
likely impact on ill-health).

5. Related to the foregoing is a need for the development of models
of the determinants (social, economic and environmental) of health
and ill health in order to provide a theoretical framework for the
empirical estimation of the effects that changes in such variables
(as well as changes in health service provision) have on health. The
current debate between advocates of prevention and those emphasizing restorative medicine, between those emphasizing wider environ-
ments and those emphasizing health services, is in urgent need of
the sort of quantification that such models, using health indicators
as outcome measures, can provide.

6. The scaling of indicators (whether they are to be on interval or
ratio scales) is a central and unresolved theoretical and empirical
question that is likely to prove divisive and an impediment to
progress unless more explicit attention is devoted to it in the future.

7. The field is pre-eminently multidisciplinary. It is one, moreover,
in which useful progress would be aided rather than inhibited by
greater collaboration across disciplinary boundaries and by more
collaboration between researchers and policy-makers.

8. The subtler philosophical, economic and political questions

concerning the role of value judgements in health indicator construction and use (whose? how aggregated? how used in social choice? and so on) are only beginning to be confronted and need substantial research.

Within each of these, more specific questions can be identified that have yet to be resolved. The workshop recognized little value in drawing up a list of detailed research 'priorities' since the priorities selected by individual researchers depend upon subjective judgements both about what is important socially and what is interesting individually. It is manifest, however, that there is a full scholarly research programme in the field and one that impinges on modern developments in many fields: psychometric measurement, epidemiology, social choice theory and ethics, medical sociology, health economics, clinical medicine.

RESEARCH ORGANIZATION

There is little value in advocating yet another brand of 'me-tooism' on behalf of the special interests of health indicators researchers. In connection with research sponsorship and organization, however, the following important conclusions should be brought to the attention of those responsible for, or influential in, research funding in general.

1. The newness of the field means that there is substantial ignorance about it and also that it may be seen by some as a kind of vague threat to an established mode of thinking, academic tradition, etc. A first priority, then, is to inform research councils, sponsors, and so on, about the nature and scope of research work in this area, its academic quality and its practical relevance.

2. The multi-disciplinary nature of the field means that existing academic disciplinary bases for research support may be inadequate to ensure the healthy continuation of this sphere of *health services* research. Moreover since much work needs to be done that is still quite remote from *immediate* policy use, the less disciplinary based policy customers of research fundings may not feel inclined to plug the resultant gap. Research councils and similar groups should therefore be aware of these difficulties and attempt an appropriate organizational response (this will involve multidisciplinary committees for the refereeing – even stimulating – of research proposals).

3. The type of research project most worthy of encouragement and support by research funding agencies is characterized by those features described above under the preceding subhead. There are, of course, also other more specific areas (for example, assessing the validity of some species of indicators) that are important substantive topics for research. These will have to be judged on the merits of the cases put up to sponsoring bodies.

4. While there are some difficulties of communication across disciplines, countries, and so on in Europe, there is in general no need for a *special* European initiative: for example a specialist journal is *not* regarded as appropriate at present. What is far more important is that research sponsors be capable of a sensitive response to research applications, and have the capability for evaluating the quality of research proposals so as to distinguish between the merely trendy and meretricious multidisciplinary proposal on the one hand and the substantial and scholarly multidisciplinary proposal on the other.

5. It is apparent that, among the European countries, Britain is the research leader in this field and has to a greater extent than elsewhere already achieved a high crossdisciplinary communication between epidemiologists, health economists, medical sociologists, psychologists, and clinicians. Communication both in Britain and Europe would be further enhanced by periodic conferences that would require finance. However, most scholars in this territory would prefer to be judged according to specific proposals about such meetings rather than make unspecific bids for resources for such purposes. It would be important, therefore, for potential sponsors to be open to the receipt of such proposals, as well as more specific proposals for substantive research. In time, the ongoing work may indicate the desirability of a European health indicators study group that would meet regularly (say once or twice a year).

6. The most productive form such a European health indicators study group could take would be as a facilitator of discussion of research proposed and in progress rather than for the presentation and discussion of finished papers of the sort most commonly presented at professional conferences. Thereby ongoing research would be subjected to greater scrutiny and (hopefully) helpful criticism than is currently the case, particularly for scholars working in relative isolation (i.e. either lacking immediate colleagues who are working on health indicators or lacking contact with scholars in the topic from other disciplines).

7. Within individual European countries there would be substantial value in establishing genuinely multidisciplinary centres of research (probably in the universities) that could pursue health indicators research either *per se* or in the wider context of health services research. Such centres should typically not be located within a single disciplinary context (for example, in medical schools) though access to such specialist departments would be necessary to enable collaborative work to be undertaken and scholarly dialogues to take place within the centres and between them and related disciplinary departments.

8. A recommendation that does not flow from the preceding discussion (and is not, indeed, central to the agenda discussed in this workshop) relates to the development of health information systems for public policy planning. Two chapters in this book (chapters 8, 9) describe in some detail the routine data available respectively in the USA and Britain and the uses to which they are and could be put. The USA has far and away the most comprehensive set of data bases available routinely. Moreover these collect data not only on aspects of health status but also on other variables that studies have shown may have a substantial impact upon it (these include not only health-service related variables but also socio-economic variables relating to income, educational attainment, race, location and many other significant correlates). Europe is a long way behind in the collection of such data and the consideration of how and in what directions European countries should be working (bearing in mind the expense of such exercises) is a central issue for researchers, clinicians and policy makers that would itself justify a workshop whose objective would be to make proposals for the development of such information systems in the contexts of European countries. Such an endeavour, devoted to the development of existing national information systems would be complementary to both the OECD work (OECD 1976) and EEC work (Armitage 1976). That is an issue to which the European Science Foundation might well direct its attention.

9. A final recommendation (but by no means the least important) is that collaborative research between social scientists on the one hand and epidemiologists and clinical researchers on the other into effectiveness and cost-effectiveness (especially under 'normal' operating conditions rather than the atypical conditions in which most researchers and enthusiasts work) be actively pursued. This territory constitutes the single most important area of ignorance we have and

is a major impediment to the rational and humane planning of health services and health policy at all levels. The development and application of health indicators in the specific context of effectiveness studies is both the highest priority and the ideal context for fruitful multidisciplinary collaborative research.

Bibliography

The following is a list of articles, books and official publications consisting of items that are either referred to in this volume or were recommended reading for some aspect of the field by a member of the workshop. To assist those who find the entire set of publications intimidating, the general bibliography is prefaced with a short list of items of article or short monograph length that were 'voted' by members of the workshop to be key items in the development of the field. The editor has exercised discretion at the margin so as to preserve a reasonable balance of discipline in the short list and to see that a representative range of application is included. A brief indication of the content of these selected items follows each. The short list is ordered temporally.

SELECTED BIBLIOGRAPHY

Katz, S., Ford, A.B., Moskowitz, R.W., Jacobson, B.A. and Jaffe, M.W. (1963) The index of ADL: A Standardised Measure of Biological and Psychosocial Function. *Journal of the American Medical Association,* **185**, 914–19.
   The Index of Activities of Daily Living encompassed six basic human functions: bathing, dressing, toileting, transfer, continence and feeding. It is a pioneering piece from which much that was neither expected nor intended has sprung.

Sullivan, D.F. (1966) *Conceptual Problems in Developing an Index of Health.* US Department of Health Education and Welfare. Publication No. (HRA) 74–1017, Series 2, No. 5, Dept. HEW, Washington D.C.
   A classic treatment of theoretical problems of constructing health indicators. A useful beginning for those seeking a pragmatic treatment of the issues.

Card, W.I. and Good, I.J. (1970) The Estimation of Implicit Utilities of Medical Consultants. *Mathematical Biosciences,* **6**, 45–54.
   An early application of the utility approach in health indicators to clinical decision-making.

Fanshel, S. and Bush, J.W. (1970) A Health Status Index and Its Application to Health Service Outcomes. *Operations Research,* **18**, 1021–66.

The classic development of the method of paired comparisons to generate weights for disability dimensions of ill-health. Indices applied to a TB screening and prevention programme.

Torrance, G.W. (1970) *A Generalized Cost-Effectiveness Model for the Evaluation of Health Programs.* Research Report Series 101, Faculty of Business, McMaster University, Hamilton.

A pioneering attempt both to develop and test various techniques for trading-off characteristics of a health indicator for use in cost-effectiveness analysis. Applied to TB care, renal failure treatment, haemolytic disease and coronary emergency care.

Culyer, A.J., Lavers, R.J. and Williams, A. (1971) Social Indicators: Health. *Social Trends,* **1**, 31–42.

The first economic interpretation of the conceptual issues underlying health indicator construction.

Patrick, D.L., Bush, J.W. and Chen, M.M. (1973) Toward an Operational Definition of Health, *Journal of Health and Social Behaviour,* **14**, 6–21.

The first application of psychometric scaling to health states and a discussion of measurement problems.

Wolfson, A.D. (1974) *A Health Index for Ontario.* Ministry of Treasury and Intergovernmental Affairs, Toronto.

The 'standard gamble' method is used to aggregate disease prevalences to identify areas of greater or lesser resource needs.

Department of Health and Human Services (1973) onwards) *Clearinghouse on Health Indexes.* US. DHHS, Hyattsville, Maryland.

Provides annual annotated bibliographies of published work on health indicators as it appears, and of ongoing research projects throughout the world.

Bergner, M., Pobbitt, R.A., Dressel, S., Pollard, W.E., Gibson, B.S. and Morris, J. (1976) The Sickness Impact Profile: Conceptual Formulations and Methodological Development of a Health Status Index. *International Journal of Health Services,* **6**, 393–415.

Development of the much-discussed Sickness Impact Profile to provide a sensitive outcome measure to guide resource allocation.

Department of Health and Social Security (1976) *Sharing Resources for Health in England,* HMSO, London.

An example of governmental use of health indicators (in this case mortality data) in the allocation of budgets to regional health authorities.

Kaplan, R.M., Bush, J.M. and Berry, C.C. (1976) Health Status: Types of Validity and the Index of Well-being. *Health Services Research,* **11**, 478–507.

The classic guide to how to validate a health index.

Organisation for Economic Cooperation and Development (1976) *Measuring Social Well-being*. OECD, Paris.
A description of the OECD social indicators programme and the place of health indicators within it.

Torrance, G.W. (1976) Towards a Utility Theory Foundation of Health Status Index Models. *Health Services Research*, **11**, 349–69.
Health status indicators are formally placed within a utility theory context and generalized. Measurement procedures are outlined.

Williams, R.G.A., Johnston, M., Willis, L.A. and Bennett, A.E. (1976) Disability: A Model and Measurement Technique. *British Journal of Preventive and Social Medicine*, **30**, 71–8.
A cumulative Guttman scale of disability is developed and validated from a community survey.

Rosser, R. and Kind, P. (1978) A Scale of Valuations of States of Illness: Is There a Social Consensus? *International Journal of Epidemiology*, 7, 347–57.
A pioneering attempt to derive a ratio scale measure of health by a structured interview instrument applied to various social and professional groups.

Wright, K.G. (1978) Output Measurement in Practice. In A.J. Culyer and K.G. Wright (eds.) *Economic Aspects of Health Services*, Martin Robertson, London.
Describes the use of Guttman scales in the measurement of the health of the elderly. The uses to which such measures may be put is discussed.

Brook, R.H., Ware, J.E., Davies-Emery, A., Stewart, A.L., Donald, C.A., Rodgers, W.H., Williams, K.N. and Johnston, S.A. (1979) *Conceptualization and Measurement of Health for Adults in the Health Insurance Study: Vol. 8, Overview*. RAND Corporation, Santa Monica.
The largest battery of health status measures ever studied.

GENERAL BIBLIOGRAPHY

Abrams, M. (1976) *A Review of Work on Subjective Social Indicators 1971–1975*. Social Science Research Council, London.

Acheson, E.D., Cowdell, R.H., Hadfield, E. and Macbeth, R.G. (1968) Nasal Cancer in Woodworkers in the furniture industry. *British Medical Journal*, ii, 587–97.

Acheson, E.D., Cowdell, R.H. and Rang, E. (1972) Adenocarcinoma of the Nasal Cavity and Sinuses in England and Wales. *British Journal of Industrial Medicine*, **29**, 21–30.

Ackerknecht, E.W. (1947) The Role of Medical History in Medical Education. *Pulletin of the History of Medicine*, **21**.

Acton, J. (1973) Discussion of Paper by Berg in Berg, B.L., *Health Status Indexes*, 147–9, Hospital Research and Education Trust, Chicago.

Ahumada, J. *et al.* (1965) *Health Planning: Problems of Concept and Method.* Publication No. 111, Pan American Health Organisation, Washington, D.C.

Aillaud, Y. (1976) *Rapport d'Activité du Centre d'Hygiène Appliquée Doria,* Marseille.

Alderson, M.R. and Whitehead, F. (1974) *Reviews of UK Statistical Sources,* Volume II, Ed. W.F. Maunder, London.

Allison, T.H. (1976) *Measuring Health Status with Local Data.* National Center for Health Statistics, 18–27.

Apple, D. (1960) How Laymen Define Illness. *Journal of Health and Human Behaviour,* 1, 219–25.

Armitage, P. (1971) *National Health Survey Systems in the EEC.* Commission of the European Communities, Luxembourg.

Armitage, P. (1976) National Health Survey Systems in the European Community. *International Journal of Epidemiology,* 5, 321–6.

Armitage, P. (1977) (ed.) *National Health Survey Systems in the European Economic Community.* Commission of the European Communities, Luxembourg.

Arrow, K.J. (1963) *Social Choice and Individual Values,* 2nd ed. Cowles Commission Monograph 12, New York, Wiley.

Auster, P. *et al.* (1972) The Production of Health: an Exploratory Study. In Fuchs 1972.

Baker, S.P., O'Neill, B., Haddon, W. and Long. W. (1974) The Injury Severity Score: A Method of Describing Patients with Multiple Injuries and Evaluating Emergency Care. *Journal of Traumatology,* 14, 187.

Balinsky, W. and Berger, R. (1975) A Review of the Research on General Health Indexes. *Medical Care,* 4.

Barlow, A. and Matthews, D. (1978) *Need for Receipt of Domiciliary Care Amongst the Elderly.* Statistics and Research Division 6, Department of Health and Social Security, London.

Barnoon, S. and Wolfe, H. (1972) *Measuring the Effectiveness of Medical Decisions: An Operations Research Approach.* Charles C. Thomas, Springfield, Illinois.

Baumann, B. (1961) Diversities in Conceptions of Health and Physical Fitness. *Journal of Health and Human Behaviour,* 3, 39–46.

Beauchamp, D. (1976) Public health as social justice. *Inquiry,* 13, 3–12.

Bebbington, A.C. (1977) Scaling Indices of Disablement. *British Journal of Preventive and Social Medicine,* 31, 122–6.

Belloc, N.B., Braslow, L. and Hochstein, J.R. (1973) Measurement of Physical Health in a General Population Survey. *American Journal of Epidemiology,* 93, 328–36.

Benson, T.J.R. (1978) Classification of Disability and Distress by Ward Nurses: A Reliability Study. *International Journal of Epidemiology,* 7, 359–61.

Beral, V. (1976) Cardiovascular Disease Mortality Trends and Oral Contraceptive Use in Young Women. *Lancet,* ii, 1047–52.

Berditt, M. and Williamson, J.W. (1973) Function Limitation Scale for Measuring Outcomes in Berg 1973b, 59–65.

Berg, O. (1975) Health and Quality of Life. *Acta Sociologica,* **18**, 3–22.

Berg, R.L. (1973a) Establishing the Values of Various Conditions of Life for a Health Status Index. In Berg 1973b, 120–7.

Berg, R.L. (1973b) *Health Status Indexes.* Hospital Research and Education Trust, Chicago.

Bergner, M., Bobbitt, R.A., Dressel, S., Pollard, W.E., Gibson, B.S. and Morris, J. (1976) The Sickness Impact Profile: Conceptual Formulations and Methodological Development of a Health Status Index. *International Journal of Health Services,* **6**, 393–415.

Bergner, M., Bobbitt, R.A., Pollard, W.E., Martin, D.P. and Gibson, B.S. (1976) The Sickness Impact Profile: Validation of a Health Status Measure. *Medical Care,* **14**, 57–67.

Bevan, G., Copeman, H., Perrin, J. and Rosser, R.M. (1980) *Health Care: Priorities and Management.* Croom Helm, London.

Bice, T.W. (1976) Comments on Health Indicators: Methodological Perspectives. *International Journal of Health Services,* **6**, 509–20.

Blaxter, M. (1976) *The Meaning of Disability.* Heinemann, London.

Blischke, W.R., Bush, J.W. and Kaplan, R.M. (1975) Successive Intervals Analysis of Preference Measures in a Health Status Index. *Health Services Research,* **10**, 181–99.

Blumstein, A. (1974) Seriousness Weights in an Index of Crime. *American Sociological Review,* **39**, 854–64.

Bond, J. and Carstairs, V. (in press) *Services for the Elderly – a Survey of the Requirements of a Population of 5000 Old People for Health and Personal Social Services.* Scottish Health Service Studies (forthcoming), Scottish Home and Health Department, Edinburgh.

Brenner, H. (1977) Health Costs and Benefits of Economic Policy. *International Journal of Health Services,* **7**, 581–623.

Brenner, H. (1979) Mortality and the National Economy. *Lancet,* **ii**, 568–73.

Breslow, L. (1972) A Quantitative Approach to the World Health Organization Definition of Health: Physical, Mental and Social Well-being. *International Journal of Epidemiology,* **1**, 347–56.

Brook, R.H., Ware, J.E., Davies-Avery, A., Stewart, A.L., Donald, C.A., Rodger, W.H., Williams, K.N. and Johnston, S.A. (1979) *Conceptualization and Measurement of Health for Adults in the Health Insurance Study, Vol. 8: Overview.* RAND Corporation, Santa Monica.

Bross, I.D.J. (1958) How to Use Ridit Analysis. *Biometrics,* **14**, 18–38.

Brun, J.P. (1975) *Approches des Bases d'une Médecine Préventive.* Universitaire de Marseille.

Bunker, J., Mosteller, C., Barnes, B. (1977) *Costs, Risks and Benefits of Surgery.* Oxford University Press, New York.

Burton, R.M., Dellinger, D.C., Dumar, W.W. and Pfeiffer, E.A. (1978) A Role for Operational Research in Health Care Planning and Management Teams. *Journal of the Operational Research Society,* **29**, 633–42.

Bush, J.W., Chen, M.M. and Patrick, D.L. (1972) Social Indicators for Health Based on Function States and Prognosis. *Proceedings of the Social Statistics Section*, American Statistical Association.

Bush, J.W., Chen, M.M., and Patrick, D.L. (1973) Health Status Index in Cost Effectiveness: Analysis of a PKU Program. In Berg 1973b, 172–94.

Bush, J.W., Chen, M.M. and Zaremba, J. (1971) Estimating Health Program Outcomes Using a Markov Equilibrium Analysis of Disease Development. *American Journal of Public Health*, 61, 2362–75.

Bush, J.W., Fanshel, S. and Chen, M.M. (1972) Analysis of a Tuberculin Testing Program Using a Health Status Index. *Socio-Economic Planning Sciences*, 6, 49.

Bush, J.W., Kaplan, R.M. and Berry, C.C. (1977) *Comparison of Methods for Measuring Social Preferences for a Health Status Index*. Annual Meeting, American Statistical Association, 682–7.

Buxton, M.J. and West, R.R. (1975) Cost-Benefit Analysis of Long-Term Haemodialysis for Chronic Renal Failure. *British Medical Journal*, ii, 376.

Cairns, J.A. (1977) *A Preliminary Report on the Use of Guttman Scaling as a Means of Constructing Dependency Categories*. Institute of Social and Economic Research, University of York.

Cairns, J.A. (1978) *Research Project on Alternative Patterns of Care for the Elderly – Interim Report*. Institute of Social and Economic Research, University of York.

Campbell, N.R. (1920) *Physics: the Elements*. (reprinted 1957) Foundations of Science, New York.

Card, W.I. (1975) *Development of a Formal Structure for Clinical Management Decisions: A Mathematical Analysis in Outcome of Severe Damage to the Central Nervous System*. Ciba Foundation Symposium 34 (New Series), Elsevier – Excerpta Medica, North Holland, Amsterdam.

Card, W.I. and Good, I.J. (1970) The Estimation of Implicit Utilities of Medical Consultants. *Mathematical Biosciences*, 6, 45–54.

Card, W.I. and Mooney, G.H. (1977) What is the Monetary Value of a Human Life? *British Medical Journal*, 11, 1627–9.

Card, W.I., Rusenkiewicz, M. and Phillips, C.I. (1977) Utility Estimates of a Set of States of Health. *Methods of Information in Medicine*, 16, 168–75.

Carley, M. (1979) Social Theory and Models in Social Indicator Research. *International Journal of Health Services*, 6, 33–54.

Carter, W.B., Bobbitt, R.A., Bergner, M. and Gibson, B.S. (1976) Validation of an Interval Scaling: The Sickness Impact Profile. *Health Services Research*, 11, 516–28.

Cayolla-da-Motta, L. (1979) A Summary Indicator of Health Status in the Municipalities and Districts of Portugal. In Holland, W.W., Ipsen, J. and Kostrzewski, J. (eds.) *Measurement of Levels of Health* (1979) 179–94.

Chambers, L.W., Sackett, D.L., Goldsmith, C.H., Macpherson, A.S. and Macauley, R.C. (1976) Development and Application of an Index of Social Function. *Health Services Research*, 11, 430–41.

Chambers, L.W., Segovia, J., Sackett, D.L., Bryant, D. and Goldsmith, C.H. (1978) *Indexes of Health. Lay and Professional Perspectives of Physical, Social and Emotional Function.* Paper to the Sociology of Health Care Session of the Learned Society Meetings, London, Ontario.

Chen, M.K. (1973) The G Index for Program Priority. In Berg 1973b, 28–34.

Chen, M.K. (1975) Alternative Estimations of Population Health Status: Further Comments and a Suggestion. *Inquiry*, **13**, 354–58.

Chen, M.K. (1976a) The K Index: A Proxy Measure of Health Care Quality. *Health Services Research*, **11**, 452–62.

Chen, M.K. (1976b) A Comprehensive Population Health Index Based on Mortality and Disability Data. *Social Indicators Research*, **3**, 257–71.

Chen, M.K. (1975) Two Forms of an Equity Index for Health Resource Allocation to Minority Groups. *Inquiry*, **13**(3), 228–32.

Chen, M.K. and Bryant, B.E. (1975) The Measurement of Health – a Critical and Selective Overview. *International Journal of Epidemiology*, **4**, 257–64.

Chen, M.M. and Bush, J.W. (1971) *A Mathematical Programming Approach for Selecting an Optimum Health Program Case Mix.* Paper to 40th National Meeting of the Operational Research Society of America, Anaheim, October.

Chen, M.M. and Bush, J.W. (1979) Health Status Measures, Policy and Biomedical Research. In Mushkin, S.J. and Dunlop, D.W. (eds.), *Health: What is it Worth? Measures of Health Benefits*, Pergamon, Oxford.

Chen, M.M., Bush, J.W. and Patrick, D.L. (1975) Social Indicators for Health Planning and Policy Analysis. *Policy Science*, **6**, 71–89.

Chen, M.M., Bush, J.W. and Zaremba, J. (1975) A Critical Analysis of Effectiveness Measures for Operations Research in Health Services in L. Schumen, J. Young, D. Speas (eds.), *Operations Research in Health – Critical Analysis*, Baltimore, John Hopkins University Press.

Chiang, C.L. (1965) *An Index of Health: Mathematical Models.* PHS Pub. No. 1000, Series 2, No. 5, U.S. Government Printing Office, Washington.

Chiang, C.L. (1976) Making Annual Indexes of Health. *Health Services Research*, **11**, 442–51.

Chiang, C.L. and Cohen, R.D. (1973) How to Measure Health: A Stochastic Model for an Index of Health. *International Journal of Epidemiology*, **2**, 7–13.

Chilton, R.J. (1969) A Review and Comparison of Simple Statistical Tests for Scalogram Analysis. *American Sociological Review*, **34**, 238–45.

Coles, J.M., Davison, A.J., Neal, D.M. and Wickings, H.I. (1976) A Comparison of Three Health Status Indicators. *International Journal of Epidemiology*, **5**, 237–46.

Committee on Medical Aspects of Automative Safety (1971) Rating the Severity of Tissue Damage I. The Abbreviated Scale. *Journal of the American Medical Association*, 215–17.

Committee on Medical Aspects of Automative Safety (1972) Rating the Severity of Tissue Damage II. The Comprehensive Injury Scale. *Journal of the American Medical Association*, 220–717.

Coombs, C.H. (1950) Psychological Scaling Without a Unit of Measurement. *Psychological Review,* 57, 145—58.

Court-Brown, W.M. and Doll, R. (1965) Mortality from Cancer and Other Causes After Radiotherapy for Ankylosing Spondilitics. *British Medical Journal,* ii, 1322—32.

Crawford, M.D., Gardner, M.J. and Morris, J.N. (1971) Cardiovascular Disease and the Mineral Content of Drinking Water. *British Medical Bulletin,* 27, 21—4.

Credoc (1966 onwards) *Comptes Nationaux de la Santé: Evaluation de la Consommation Medicale,* Paris.

Cullen, M.J. (1975) *The Statistical Movement in Early Victorian Britain.* Harvester Press, New York.

Culyer, A.J. (1972a) Appraising Government Expenditure on Social Services: The Problems of 'need' and 'output'. *Public Finance,* 27, 205—11.

Culyer, A.J. (1972b) Indicators of Health: An Economist's Viewpoint. In *Evaluation in the Health Services,* Office of Health Economics, London.

Culyer, A.J. (1978) *Measuring Health: Lessons for Ontario,* Toronto University Press, Toronto.

Culyer, A.J. (1978) Need, Values and Health Status Measurement. In Culyer and Wright 1978, 9—31.

Culyer, A.J. (1979) What Do Health Services Do for People? *Search,* 10, 262—8.

Culyer, A.J. (1980) *The Political Economy of Social Policy.* Martin Robertson, Oxford.

Culyer, A.J., Lavers, R.J. and Williams, A. (1971) Social Indicators: Health. *Social Trends,* 1, 31—42. Her Majesty's Stationery Office.

Culyer, A.J., Lavers, R.J. and Williams, A. (1972) Health Indicators in *Social Indicators and Social Policy.* Ed. Shonfield, A. and Shaw, S., Heinemann, London.

Culyer, A.J. and Simpson, H. (1980) Externality Models and Health: a Ruckblick Over the Last Twenty Years. *Economic Record,* 56, 222—30.

Culyer, A.J. and Wright, K.G. (1978) *Economic Aspects of Health Services,* Martin Robertson, Oxford.

Culyer, A.J. (1976) *Need and the National Health Service,* Martin Robertson, London.

Dahlstrom, W.G. and Welsh, G.S. (1960) *MMPI Handbook: A Guide to Use in Clinical Practice and Research.* University of Minnesota Press, Minneapolis.

Dalkey, N. (1969a) Analyses from a Group Opinion Study. *Futures,* 1, 408.

Dalkey, N. (1969b) Analyses from a Group Opinion Study. *Futures,* 1, 541.

Damiani, P. (1973) La Mesure du Niveau de Santé. *Journal de la Société de Statistique de Paris,* 2, 129—44.

Dawson, W.E. and Mirando, M.A. (1976) Inverse Scales of Opinion Obtained by Sensory-Modality Matching. *Perceptual and Motor Skills,* 42, 415—25.

Delaroche, J.P. (1979) *La Distribution des Risques dans un Groupe Humain,* Universitaire de Paris XI.

Dembrowsky, T.M. *et al.* (1978) (ed.) *Coronary Prone Behaviour*. Springer, New York.

Department of Health Education and Welfare (1976) *Health Planning Information Series: Guide for Health Systems Planners*, DHEW Publication No. 76–1450, US Government Printing Office, Washington D.C.

Department of Health Education and Welfare (1979) *Health Statistics Plan. Fiscal Years 1979–80*, Public Health Service, Washington D.C.

Department of Health and Human Services (1973 onwards) *Clearinghouse on Health Indexes: Cumulated Annotations*, US DHHS, Hyattsville, Maryland.

Department of Health and Human Services (1980) *Health–United States: 1980*. Hyattsville, Maryland: DHHS Publication No. (PHS) 81–1232, US DHHS, Washington D.C.

Department of Health and Social Security (1976) *Sharing Resources for Health in England*, HMSO, London.

Department of Health and Social Security (1980) *Inequalities in Health*. DHSS, London.

Department of Operational Research of University of Lancaster (1968) *Patrol Effectiveness and Patrol Deployment*. Report to the Home Office.

Dingle, H. (1950) A Theory of Measurement. *British Journal of Philosophy and Science*, 1, 5–26.

Doherty, N. and Hicks, D. (1977) Cost-Effectiveness and Alternative Health Care Programs for the Elderly. *Health Services Research*, 12, 190–203.

Doll, R. and Hill, A.B. (1964) Mortality in Relation to Smoking: Ten Years' Observation of British Doctors. *British Medical Journal*, 1399–1410.

Donnan, S. and Haskey, J. (1977) Alcoholism and Cirrhosis of the Liver. *Population Trends*, 7, 18–24.

Douglas, J. (1967) *The Social Meaning of Suicide*. Princeton University Press, Princeton.

Draper, J. (1963) A Suggested Method for Constructing Indices of Morbidity. *Applied Statistics*, 3, 26–37.

Dublin, L.I. and Lotka, A.J. (1930) *The Money Value of a Man*. Ronald Press, New York.

Duckett, S.J. and Kristofferson, S.M. (1978) An Index of Hospital Performance. *Medical Care*, 16, 400–7.

Eisler, H. (1962) On the Problems of Category Scales in Psychophysics. *Scandinavian Journal of Psychology*, 3, 81–7.

Ekman, G. (1962) Measurement of Moral Judgement: A Comparison of Scaling Methods. *Perceptual and Motor Skills*, 15, 3–9.

Elinson, J. (1980) Medical Sociology: Theoretical Underdevelopment and Some Opportunities. In Blalock, H.M. (ed.) *Sociological Theory and Research*, Free Press, New York, pp. 373–81.

Ellis, B. (1966) *Basic Concepts of Measurement*. Cambridge University Press.

v. Engelhardt, D. (1978) *Normalitat und Krankheit*, STE 2, Funkkolleg Umwelt und Gesundheit, Weinheim.

Eyer, J. (1977) Does Unemployment Cause the Death Rate Peak in Each Business Cycle? A Multifactorial Model of Death Rate Change. *International Journal of Health Services*, 7, 625–62.

Fanshel, S. (1972) A Meaningful Measure of Health for Epidemiology. *International Journal of Epidemiology*, 1, 319–37.

Fanshel, S. and Bush, J.W. (1970) A Health Status Index and its Application to Health Service Outcomes. *Operations Research*, 18, 1021–66.

Fechner, G.T. (1907) *Elemente der Psychophysik*, Preitkopf and Hartel, Leipzig.

v. Ferber, C. (1978a) Gesundheit und Krankheit im Wandel der Gesellschaft. In: Ferber and Ferber (1978).

v. Ferber, C. (1978b) Zur Gesundheitspolitik in der Bundesrepublik. In Ferber and Ferber (1978).

v. Ferber, C. and v. Ferber, L. (1978) *Der Kranke Mensch in der Gesellschaft*, Hamburg.

v. Ferber, L. (1978) Arzt-Patient-Beziehung. In Ferber and Ferber (1978).

Field, D. (1976) The Social Definition of Illness. In Tuckett (1976).

Fisher, I. (1909) Report on National Vitality: Its Wastes and Conservation. *Bulletin of One Hundred on National Health*, No. 30, Washington D.C.

Forst, B.E. (1973) Quantifying the Patient's Preferences. In Berg (1973b), 209–21.

Fox, A.J. (1977) Occupational Mortality 1970–72. *Population Trends*, 9, 8–15.

Fox, A.J. (1980) Prospects for Measuring Changes in Differential Mortality. In *Proceedings of a meeting in Mexico City on Socio-economic determinants and consequences of differential mortality*, WHO, Geneva.

Fox, A.J. (1981a) Design Problems and Data Collection Strategies in Studies of Mortality Differentials in Developed Countries. *International Union for Scientific Study of Population Conference in Senegal*, July 1981.

Fox, A.J. (1981b) *Recent Developments in Mortality and Cancer Statistics. Proceedings of 1980 Statistics Users' Conference.* (In press).

Fox, A.J. and Goldblatt, P.O. (1982) *Socio-Demographic Mortality Differentials: OPCS Longitudinal Study 1971–75*, Series L5, No. 1, HMSO, London.

Fuchs, V. (1972) *Essays in the Economics of Health and Medical Care*, National Bureau of Economic Research, New York.

Fuchs, V. (1979) The Economics of Health in the Post-Industrial Society, *Public Interest*, 56 Summer, 3–20.

Gadreau, M. (1976) *Contribution à la Planification des Actions de Santé*, Université de Dijon, Dijon.

Garcia, A.M. (1976) Problems in the Ratio Measurement of Life Stress. *Journal of Health and Social Behaviour*, 17, 70–82.

Garrad, J. (1974) Impairment and Disability: their Measurement, Prevalence and Psychological Cost. in Lees, D. and Shaw, S. (eds.), *Impairment, Disability and Handicap*, 141–56, Heinemann, London.

Garrad, J. and Bennett, A.E. (1971) A Validated Interview Schedule for Use in

Population Surveys of Chronic Disease Disability. *British Journal of Preventive and Social Medicine*, **25**, 97–104.

Gibbs, R.J. (1970) *Crime Seriousness: A Review of the Literature in Relation to Possible Police Use*. Home Office Planning Organisation Report No. 12/70 (Unpublished).

Gibbs, R.J. (1972) *A Scale of Crime Seriousness for Police Use*. Home Office Police Planning Organisation Report. No. 10/72.

Gibbs, R.J. (1974) *Performance Measures in Public Services*. Ph.D. Thesis, University of Warwick.

Gibson, B.S., Gibson, J.S., Bergner, M., Bobbitt, B.A., Kressel, S., Pollard, W.E. and Vesselage, M. (1975) The Sickness Impact Profile. *American Journal of Public Health*, **65**.

Goldberg, M. (1978) *Mesure de l'Etat de Santé*. Document de travail du GERSS, Paris.

Goldberg, M., Dab, W., Chaperon, J., Fuhrer, R., Gremy, F. (1979) Indicateurs de Santé et "Sanometrie": les Aspects Conceptuels des Recherches Recentes sur la Mesure de L'état de Santé d'une Population. *Revue Epidemiologic et Santé*, 27, 51–68 and 133–152.

Goldblatt, P. (personal communication to A.J. Fox).

Goldsmith, S.B. (1972) The Status of Health States Indicators. *Health Services Reports*, 87, 212–20.

Grogono, A.W. and Woodgate, D.J. (1971) Index for Measuring Health. *Lancet*, ii, 1024–6.

Grossman, M. (1972) *The Demand for Health: A Theoretical and Empirical Investigation*. Columbia University Press, New York.

Gustafson, D.H. and Holloway, D.C. (1975) A Decision Theory Approach to Measuring Severity of Illness. *Health Services Research*, Spring, 97–106.

Hagard, S., Carter, F. and Milne, R.G. (1976) Screening for Spina Bifida Cystica. *British Journal of Preventive and Social Medicine*, 30, 40.

Harris, A.I. (1971) *Handicapped and Impaired in Great Britain*. HMSO, London.

Harris, G. (1979) *Planning Systems and the Allocation of Resources: Decentralised Planning in the National Health Service*. Unpublished Mimeo, DHSS, London.

Heady, J.A. and Heasman, M.A. (1959) *Social and Biological Factors in Infant Mortality*. Studies in Medical and Population Subjects. No. 15, HMSO, London.

Health Statistics in Britain (in press) *Proceedings of the 1980 Statistics Users Conference held at the Royal Society, December 1980*.

Henke, K.-b. (1975) *Die Verteilung von Guetern und Diensten auf die verschiedenen Bevoelkerungsschichten*, Schwartz, Goettingen.

Henke, K.-D. (1977) Oeffentliche Gesundheitsausgaben und Verteilung, Vandenhoeck and Ruprecht, Goettingen.

Hightower, W.L. (1978) Development of an Index of Health Utilising Factor Analysis. *Medical Care*, **16**, 245–55.

Hindelang, M.J. (1974) The Uniform Crime Reports Revisited. *Journal of Criminal Justice*, 2, 1–17.

Holland, W., Ipsen, J. and Kostrzewski, J. (1979) Eds. *Measurement of Levels of Health*, World Health Organisation, Geneva.

Holmes, T.H. and Rahe, R.H. (1967) The Social Re-Adjustment Rating Scale. *Journal of Psychosomatic Research*, 11, 213–18.

Holloway, D.C. (1973) Evaluating Health States for Utilisation. In Berg (1973b), 89–98.

Home Office (1978) *Report of the Committee on Data Protection*. HMSO, London.

Hough, R.L., Fairbank, D.T. and Garcia, A.M. (1976) Problems in the Ratio Measurement of Life Stress. *Journal of Health and Social Behaviour*, 17, 70–82.

Hull, J., Moore, P.G., and Thomas, H. (1973) Utility and Its Measurement. *Journal of the Royal Statistical Society*, 136, 226–47.

Hunt, S.M. and McEwen, J. (1980) The Development of a Subjective Health Indicator. *Sociology of Health and Illness*, 2, 231–46.

Hunter, D.J. (1979) Practice: Decisions and Resources in the National Health Service (Scotland). In *The Ethics of Resource Allocation in Health Care*, ed. K.M. Boyd, Edinburgh University.

Illsley, R. (1977) Everybody's Business? Concepts of Health and Illness. In: Social Science Research Council, *Health and health policy priorities for research*, Social Science Research Council, London.

Inman, W.H.W. (1981a) Postmarketing Surveillance of Adverse Drug Reactions in General Practice: I Search for New Methods. *British Medical Journal*, 282, 1131–2.

Inman, W.H.W. (1981b) Postmarketing Surveillance of Adverse Drug Reactions in General Practice: II Prescription-event Monitoring at the University of Southampton. *British Medical Journal*, 282, 1216–17.

Inman, W.H.W. and Adelstein, A.M. (1969) Rise and Fall of Asthma Mortality in England and Wales in Relation to the Use of Pressurised Aerosols. *Lancet*, ii, 279–85.

Isaacs, B., Livingston, M. and Neville, Y. (1972) *Survival of the Unfittest*, Routledge, London.

Jacquet-Lagreze, E. (1979) De la Logique d'Agrégation des Criteres à une Logique d'Agrégation-Desagrégation des Préférences. *Economie et Société*, 6, 839–58.

Jazairi, N.T. (1976) *Approaches to the Development of Health Indicators*. OECD Special Studies No. 2, OECD Social Indicator Development Programme, Paris.

Jefferys, M., Millard, J.B., Hyman, M. and Warren, M.D. (1969) A Set of Tests for Measuring Motor Impairment in Prevalence Studies. *Journal of Chronic Diseases*, 22, 303–19.

Jenicek, M., Rousseau, T. and Bellefleur, M. (1977) Santé Physique Mentale, Sociale et Handicaps de Citoyens Seniors, Ville de Saint-Laurent – II Sante Globale, Incapacité et Dependance. *Canadian Journal of Public Health,* **68**, 323–9.

Johnson, M.L. (1972) Self-perception of Need Amongst the Elderly: An Analysis of Illness Behaviour. *Sociological Review,* **20**, 521–31.

Johnston, D. (1977) *Basic Disaggregations of Main Social Indicators,* Special Studies No. 4, OECD Social Indicator Development Programme, Paris.

Kaplan, A. (1964) *The Conduct of Inquiry.* Chandler, San Francisco.

Kaplan, R.M., Bush, J.W. and Berry, C.C. (1976) Health Status: Types of Validity and the Index of Well-Being. *Health Services Research,* **11**, 478–507.

Kaplan, R.M., Bush, J.W. and Berry, C.C. (1979) Health Status Index: Category Rating Versus Magnitude Estimation for Measuring Levels of Well-Being. *Medical Care,* **17**, 501–25.

Katz, S. and Akpom, C.A. (1976) A Measure of Primary Socio-Biological Functions. *International Journal of Health Services,* **6**.

Katz, S., Akpom, C.A., Papsidero, J.A. and Weiss, S.T. (1973) Measuring the Health Status of Populations. In Berg (1973b), 39–51.

Katz, S., Downs, T.D., Cash, H.R. and Grotz, R.C. (1970) Progress in Development of the Index of ADL. *Gerontology,* **10**, 20.

Katz, S., Ford, A.B., Chinn, A.B. and Newill, V.A. (1966) Prognosis After Strokes: Long Term Course of 159 Patients. *Medicine,* **45**, 236.

Katz, S., Ford, A.B., Heiple, K.G. and Newill, V.A. (1964) Studies of Illness in the Aged: Recovery After Fracture of the Hip. *Journal of Gerontology,* **19**, 285.

Katz, S., Ford, A.B., Moskowitz, R.W., Jacobson, B.A. and Jaffe, M.W. (1963) The Index of ADL: A Standardised Measure of Biological and Psychosocial Function. *Journal of the American Medical Association,* **185**, 914–19.

Katz, S., Vignos, P.J., Moskowitz, R.W., Thompson, H.M. and Svec, K.H. (1968) Comprehensive Outpatient Care in Rheumatoid Arthritis: A Controlled Study. *Journal of the American Medical Association,* **206**, 1249.

Kind, P. and Rosser, R.M. (1980a) Ratio and Interval Scales from the Same Psychometric Data. In Rosser (1980).

Kind, P. and Rosser, R.M. (1980b) *Health Indicators: Sensitivity and Robustness.* Presented at the 2nd International Conference on Systems Science in Health Care, Montreal, July 1980, Pergamon, (in press).

Kind, P., Rosser, R.M. and Williams, A. (1981) *Valuation of the Quality of Life: Some Psychometric Evidence.* Presented at the Geneva Conference on the Value of Life and Safety, organised by the Association Internationale pour l'Etude de l'Economie de l'Assurance. 30 March–1 April 1981.

Kind, P. (1981) *A Comparison of Two Models for Scaling Health Indicators.* To be submitted for publication.

Kirkpatrick, J. and Youmans, R. (1971) Trauma Index: An Aid in the Evaluation of Injury Victims. *Journal of Traumatology,* **11**, 711.

Kisch, A.I., Karner, H.W., Harris, L.J. and Kline, G. (1969) A New Proxy Measure for Health Status. *Health Services Research*, 4, 223–30.

Kneppreth, N.P., Gustafsen, D.H., Rose, J.H. and Leifer, R.P. (1973) Techniques for the Assessment of Worth. In Berg (1973b), 228–38.

Kosa, J. and Robertson, L. (1969) The Social Aspects of Health and Illness. In J. Kosa, A. Antonovsky and I. Zola (eds.) *Poverty and Health*, Harvard University Press, Cambridge Mass.

Krantz, D.H. (1972) A Theory of Magnitude Estimation and Cross-Modality Matching. *Journal of Mathematical Psychology*, 9, 169–99.

Krischer, J.P. (1976) Indexes of Severity: Underlying Concepts. *Health Services Research*, 11, 143–57.

Lawton, M.P., Ward, M. and Yaffer, S. (1967) Indices of Health in an Aging Population. *Journal of Gerontology*, 22, 334–42.

Levine, D.S. and Yett, D.E. (1973) A Method for Constructing Proxy Measures of Health Status. In Berg (1973b), 12–22.

Levy, E. (1974) Health Indicators and Health Systems Analysis. In M. Perlman (ed.), *The Economics of Health and Medical Care*, Macmillan, London.

Linn, B.S., Linn, M.W. and Gurel, L. (1968) Cumulative Illness Rating Scale. *Journal of the American Geriatric Society*, 16, 622.

Linn, M.W. (1967) A Rapid Disability Rating Scale. *Journal of the American Geriatric Society*, 15, 211–14.

Linn, M.W., Gurel, L. and Linn, B.S. (1977) Patient Outcome as a Measure of Quality of Nursing Care. *American Journal of Public Health*, 67, 337–44.

Logan, W.P.D. and Brooke, E.M. (1957) *The Survey of Sickness 1943 to 1952*. General Register Office, Studies on Medical and Population Subjects No. 12, HMSO, London.

Luce, R.D. (1972) What Sort of Measurement is Psychophysical Measurement? *American Psychologist*, 27, 96–106.

Lueth, P. (1979) *Das Krankheitenbuch*, Darmstadt.

McFadden, D. (1975) The Revealed Preference of a Government Bureaucracy: Theory. *Bell Journal of Economics*, 6, 401.

MacFarlane, A. (1977) Daily Mortality and Environment in English Connurbations I: Air Pollution, Low Temperature and Influenza in Greater London. *British Journal of Preventive and Social Medicine*, 31, 54–61.

McKenna, S.P., Hunt, S.M. and McEwen, J. (1981) Weighting the Seriousness of Perceived Health Problems Using Thurstone's Method of Paired Comparisons. *International Journal of Epidemiology*, 10, 93–7.

McKeown, T. (1976) *The Role of Medicine: Dream, Mirage, or Nemises?* Nuffield Provincial Hospitals Trust, London.

McKeown, T. (1980) *The Role of Medicine: Dream Mirage, or Nemesis?* (Second edition). Blackwell, Oxford.

McKinlay, J. and McKinlay, S. (1972) Some Characteristics of Lower Working Class Utilizers and Under Utilizers of the Maternity Services. *Journal of Health and Social Behaviour*, 13, 369–82.

McNeil, B., Weichselbaum, R., Pauker, S.G. (1978) Fallacy of the Five Year Survival in Lung Cancer. *New England Journal of Medicine,* 299, 1879–1401.

Maddox, G.L. (1964) Self-Assessment of Health Status – A Longitudinal Study of Elderly Subjects. *Journal of Chronic Diseases,* 17, 449–60.

Maddox, G.L. (1972) Interventions and Outcomes: Notes on Designing and Implementing an Experiment in Health Care. *International Journal of Epidemiology,* 1, 339–47.

Magdelaine, M., Misrahi, A., and Rosch, G. (1967) Un Indicateur de la Morbidité Appliqué aux Données d'une Enquête sur la Consommation Medicale. *Consommation, Annales du C.R.E.D.O.C. Centre de Recherches et de Documentation sur la Consommation,* 2, 3–41.

Martini, C.J.M., Allan, G.J.B., Davison, J. and Backett, E.M. (1979) Health Indexes Sensitive to Medical Care Variation. In J. Elinson and A. Siegmann (eds.), *Socio-medical Health Indicators,* Baywood, Farmingdale, pp. 145–154.

Martini, C.J. and McDowell, I. (1976) Health Status: Patient and Physician Judgements. *Health Services Research,* Winter, 508–15.

Masuda, M. and Holmes, T.H. (1967) Magnitude Estimations of Social Readjustments. *Journal of Psychosomatic Research,* 1, 219–26.

Maxwell, R.J. (1981) *Health and Wealth: An International Study of Health Care Spending.* Lexington Books, Lexington.

Mead, M. (1950) *Sex and Temperament in Three Primitive Societies,* New York, Mentor.

Mechanic, D. (1968) *Medical Sociology.* The Free Press, New York.

Menrad, J. and Colvez, A. (1978) Etude d'un Indicateur de Santé Destiné a l'Evaluation de l'Efficacité d'une Consultation Exterue. *Santé Publique,* 26, 391–402.

Miller, J.E. (1973) Guidelines for Selecting a Health Status Index: Suggested Criteria. In Berg (1973b), 243–7.

Miller, J.E. (1970) An Indicator to Aid Management in Assigning Program Priorities. *Public Health Reports,* 85, 725.

Mishan, E.J. (1972) *Cost-Benefit Analysis.* George Allen and Unwin, London.

Mizrahi, A., Mizrahi, A. and Rosch, G. (1973) Un Indicateur de Morbidité. *Consommation,* 2, 7–55.

Mooney, G.H. (1977) *The Valuation of Human Life.* Macmillan, Basingstoke.

Morley, R. (1972) Comment on the Implicit Valuation of Forms of Hospital Treatment. In M.M. Hauser (ed.) *The Economics of Medical Care,* George Allen and Unwin Ltd. London.

Moriyama, I.W. (1968) Problems in the Measurement of Health Status. In Sheldon, E.B. and Moore, W.E. *Indicators of Social Change,* 573–600. Russell Sage Foundation, New York.

National Center for Health Statistics (1965) *Vital and Health Statistics,* Series 1, No. 4: Plan and Initial Programme of the Health Examination Survey, Washington D.C.

National Center for Health Statistics (1977) Statistics Needed for Determining the Effects of the Environment on Health. *Vital and Health Statistics*, Publication No. (PHS 79–1457), Series 4, No. 20, Public Health Service, Hyattsville, Maryland.

National Center for Health Statistics (1979) *Health US*. NCHS, Hyattsville, Maryland.

Neumann, J. von and Morgenstern, O. (1947) *Theory of Games and Economic Behaviour*. (2nd ed.), Princeton University Press, Princeton.

Nishi, S. (1971) The Development of Health Status Indicators in Japan for Health Planning. *Bulletin of the Institute of Public Health, Tokyo*, 20, 62–77.

Nunally, J.C. and Durham, R.L. (1975) Validity, Reliability and Special Problems of Measurement in Evaluation Research. In Strieenig and Guttentag (1975).

Nunally, J.C. and Durham, R.L. (1975) Method and Theory for Developing Measures in Evaluation Research. In Strieenig and Guttentag (1975).

Nuyens, Y. (1977) Health Indicators. In Armitage (1977).

Office of Federal Statistical Policy and Standards (1978) *A Framework for Planning US Federal Statistics for the 1980's*, US Dept. of Commerce, Washington D.C.

Office of Population Censuses and Surveys (1978a) *Occupational Mortality 1970–72*. Decennial Supplement, DS No. 1, HMSO, London.

Office of Population Censuses and Surveys (1978b) *Trends in Mortality 1951–75*. DH1 No. 3, HMSO, London.

Office of Population Censuses and Surveys (1980a) *Cancer Statistics (Survival) 1971–73*. MB1 No. 3, HMSO, London.

Office of Population Censuses and Surveys (1981b) *Mortality Surveillance 1968–77*. (unpublished).

Office of Technology Assessment (1979) *Selected Topics in Federal Health Statistics*, OTA, Congress of the US, Washington D.C.

Organisation for Economic Cooperation and Development (1974) *Social Indicators – the OECD Experience*. OECD, Paris.

Organisation for Economic Cooperation and Development (1976) *Measuring Social Well-Being*. OECD, Paris.

Organisation for Economic Cooperation and Development (1977) *Public Expenditures on Health*. OECD, Paris.

Packer, A.H. (1968) Applying Cost-Effectiveness Concepts to the Community Health System. *Operations Research*, 16, 227–53.

Parsons, T. (1951) *The Social System*. Free Press, New York.

Parsons, T. (1972) Definitions of Health and Illness in the Light of American Values and Social Structure. In E.G. Jaco (ed.), *Patients, Physicians and Illness* (Second edition). Free Press, New York, pp. 107–127.

Patrick, D.L. (1976) Constructing Social Matrices for Health Status Indexes. *International Journal of Health Services*, 6, 443–53.

Patrick, D.L. (1979) Constructing Social Metrics for Health Status Indexes. In J. Elinson and A. Siegmann (eds.), *Socio-medical Health Indicators*, Baywood, Farmingdale.

Patrick, D.L., Bush, J.W. and Chen, M.M. (1973a) Towards an Operational Definition of Health. *Journal of Health and Social Behaviour*, 14, 6–21.

Patrick, D.L., Bush, J.W. and Chen, M.M. (1973b) Methods for Measuring Levels of Well-Being for a Health Status Index. *Health Services Research*, 8, 229–44.

Patrick, D.L., Darby, S., Green, S., Horton, G., Locker, D. and Wiggins, R. (in press) Screening for Disability in the Inner City. *Epidemiology and Community Health*, (forthcoming).

Paykel, E.S. (1974) Recent Life Events and Clinical Depression. In Gunderson, E.K.E., and Rahe, R.H. (eds.) *Life Stress and Illness*, Thomas, Springfield, Illinois.

Plishkin, J.S. and Beck, C.H. (1976) A Health Index for Patient Selection: A Value Function Approach with Application to Chronic Renal Failure Patients, *Management Science*, 22, 1009–21.

Pollard, W.E., Bobbitt, R.A., Bergner, M., Martin, D.P. and Gibson, B.S. (1976) The Sickness Impact Profile. Reliability of a Health Status Measure. *Medical Care*, 14.

Querido, A. (1963) *The Efficiency of Medical Care*. Leiden, Stanfert Kroese.

Raiffa, H. (1968) *Decision Analysis*. Addison-Wesley, Reading, Mass.

Redfern, P. (1976) *Office of Population Censuses and Surveys, Population Trends*, No. 4, 21–3.

Reid, D.D. (1969) The Beginnings of Bronchitis. *Proceedings of Royal Society of Medicine*, 62, 1–6.

Reid, D.D. (1975) International Studies in Epidemiology. *American Journal of Epidemiology*, 102, 469–76.

Reynolds, W.J., Rushing, W.A. and Miles, D.L. (1974) The Validation of a Function Status Index. *Journal of Health and Social Behaviour*, 15, 271–89.

Rippere, V. (1976) Scaling the Seriousness of Illness: A Methodological Study. *Journal of Psychosomatic Research*, 20, 567–73.

Roemer, M.I., Moustafa, A.T. and Hopkins, C.E. (1968) A Proposed Hospital Quality Index: Hospital Death Rates Adjusted for Case Severity. *Health Services Research*, 3, 96–119.

Romano, J. (1950) Basic Orientation and Education of the Medical Student. *Journal of the American Medical Association*, 143, 409–12.

Rosch, G. (1976) La Taxonomie Nosologique. *Consommation*, 22, 5–36.

Rose, G. (1966) Cold Weather and Ischaemic Heart Disease. *British Journal of Preventive and Social Medicine*, 20, 97–100.

Rosser, R.M. (1974) *The Measurement of Hospital Output – A Case Study*. Paper to the Royal Society of Health Congress. Published in the Proceedings, pp. 88–92.

Rosser, R.M. (1976) Recent Studies Using a Gobal Approach to Measuring Illness. *Medical Care Supplement*, **14**, 138—47.

Rosser, R.M. (1977) Health Status Indicators. *International Journal of Epidemiology*, **6**, 89—90.

Rosser, R.M. (1980) *A Set of Descriptions and a Psychometric Scale of Severity of Illness: An Indicator for Use in Evaluating the Outcome of Hospital Care*. Ph.D. Thesis, University of London, Chapters 7 and 8.

Rosser, R.M. (1981) Life with Artificial Organs — Renal Dialysis and Transplants. In *Personal Meanings*, Eds. E. Shepherd and J. Watson, to be published by John Wiley and Sons, Chicester.

Rosser, R.M. and Benson, T.J.R. (1978) New Tools for Evaluation: Their Application to Computers. In *Lecturer Notes on Medical Informatics*, 1, Medical Informatics Europe 78, ed. Andersen, J., Springer-Verlag, 701—10.

Rosser, R.M. and Kind, P. (1978) A Scale of Valuations of States of Illness: Is There a Social Consensus? *International Journal of Epidemiology*, **7**, 347—57.

Rosser, R.M. and Watts, V.C. (1971) *The Sanative Output of a Hospital*. Paper to the 39th Operational Research Society of America, Dallas.

Rosser, R.M. and Watts, V.C. (1972) The Measurement of Hospital Output. *International Journal of Epidemiology*, **1**, 361—7.

Rosser, R.M. and Watts, V.C. (1973) The Development of a Classification of the Symptoms of Sickness. In Lees, D. and Shaw, S. (eds.), *Impairmen, Disability and Handicap*, Heinemann, London.

Rosser, R.M. and Watts, V.C. (1975) Disability — A Clinical Classification. *New Law Journal*, **125**, 323—5.

Rosser, R.M. and Watts, V.C. (1976) An Operational Objective for Health Services. *Proceedings of the Conference of the European Federation of Operational Research Societies*, (Euro II), Stockholm.

Rosser, R.M. and Watts, V.C. (1977a) Do Patients Get Better in Hospital? In Barber, B. *Selected Papers on Operational Research in the Health Services*, 68—87, The Operational Research Society.

Rosser, R.M. and Watts, V.C. (1977b) Measurement of the Effectiveness of Health Services, *Proceedings of International Congress on Computing in Medicine*, (Med. Comp. 77) Berlin.

Rosser, R.M. and Watts, V.C. (1978) The Measurement of Illness. *Journal of Operational Research*, **29**, 529—40.

Royal Society Working Party on the Assessment and Perception of Risk (1983a) *Report of Sub-group on Epidemiological Methods of Assessing Risks to Man*.

Royal Society Working Party on the Assessment and Perception of Risk (1983b) *Report of Sub-group on Use of Laboratory Methods of Assessing Risks to Man*.

Royal Society Working Party on the Assessment and Perception of Risk (1983c) *Report of Sub-group on Risk Management*.

Russell, B. (1938) *Principles of Mathematics*, Second Ed. Horton, New York.

Sackett, D.L. (with 12 others) (1974) The Burlington Randomised Trial of the Nurse Practitioner: Health Outcomes of Patients. *Annals of Internal Medicine*, **80**, 137.

Sackett, D.L., Chambers, L.W., MacPherson, A.S., Goldsmith, C.H. and Macauley, R.G. (1977) The Development and Application of Indices of Health: General Methods and a Summary of Results. *American Journal of Public Health*, **67**, 423–7.

Sackett, D.L. and Torrance, G.W. (1978) The Utility of Different Health States as Perceived by the General Public. *Journal of Chronic Diseases*, **31**, 697–704.

Sainsbury, S. (1970) *Registered as Disabled*. Occasional papers in social administration, No. 35, Bell, London.

Sainsbury, S. (1973) *Measuring Disability*. Occasional papers in social administration, No. 54, Bell, London.

Samuelson, P.A. (1948) Consumption Theory in Terms of Revealed Preference, *Economica*, 243.

Sanders, B.S. (1964) Measuring Community Health Levels. *American Journal of Public Health*, **54**, 1063–70.

Savage, C.W. (1970) *The Measurement of Sensation*. University of California Press.

Schaefer, H. (1976) Der Krankheitsbegriff. *Handbuch der Sociolmedizin*, **3**, 15.

Schaefer, H. (1978) *Umwelt und Gesundheit*, STE 1, Funkkolleg Umwelt und Gesundheit, Weinheim.

Schaefer, H. and Schipperges, H. (1978) *Gesundheitserziehung*. STE 18, Funkkolleg Umwelt und Gesundheit, Weinheim.

Scheffler, R.M. and Lipscomb, J. (1974) Alternative Estimations of Population Health Status: an Empirical Example. *Inquiry*, **11**, 220–8.

Sellin, T. and Wolfgang, M. (1964) *The Measurement of Delinquency*. Wiley, New York.

Siegmann, A.E. (1976) A Classification of Socio-Medical Health Indicators: Prospectives for Health Administrative and Health Planners. *International Journal of Health Services*, **6**.

Siegrist, J. (1977) *Lehrbuch der Medizinischen Soziologie*. Urbahn and Schwarzenberg, München.

Scottish Home and Health Dept. (1977) *Scottish Health Authorities Revenue Equalisation*, HMSO, Edinburgh.

Siegrist, J. *et al.* (1980) *Soziale Belastungen und Herzinfarkt*. Enke, Stuttgart.

Siegerist, H.E. (1960) *On the Sociology of Medicine*. (ed.) Roemer, M.I., Lo-11, MD Publications Inc., New York.

Skinner, D.E. and Yett, D.E. (1973) Debility Index for Long-term Care Patients. In Berg (1973b), 69–82.

Spautz, M.E. (1972) The Socio-Economic Gap. *Socio-Economic Research*, **1**, 211–29.

Stacey, M. (1977) Concepts of Health and Illness: A Working Paper on the Concepts and Their Relevance for Research. In *Health and Health Policy*, Report of an Advisory Panel to the Research Initiatives Board, London,

Social Science Research Council.

Starfield, B. (1973) Health Services Research: a Working Model. New England *Journal of Medicine*, **289**, 132.

Starfield, B. (1974) Measurement of Outcome: a Proposed Scheme. *Health and Society*, Winter, 39–49.

Stevens, J.C., Mark, J.D. and Stevens, S.S. (1960) Growth of Sensation of Seven Continua as Measured by Force of Handgrip. *Journal of Experimental Psychology*, **59**, 60–7.

Stevens, S.S. (1946) On the Theory of Scales of Measurement. *Science*, **103**, 677–80.

Stevens, S.S. (1959a) Measurement, Psychophysics and Utility. In Churchman, C.W. and Ratoosh, P. *Measurement, Definitions and Theories*, Wiley, New York, pp. 18–63.

Stevens, S.S. (1959b) Cross-Modality Validation of Subjective Scales for Loudness, Vibration and Electric Shock. *Journal of Experimental Psychology*, **57**, 201–209.

Stevens, S.S. (1960) Ratio, Partition and Confusion Scales. In *Psychological Scaling: Theory and Applications*, (eds.), Gulliksen, H. and Messick, S., Wiley, New York.

Stevens, S.S. (1964) Matching Functions Between Loudness and Ten Other Continua. *Perception and Psychophysics*, **1**, 5–7.

Stevens, S.S. (1966) A Metric for the Social Consensus. *Science*, **151**, 530–41.

Steward, A., Ware, J.F., Brook, R.H. and Davies-Avery, A. (1978) *A Conceptualization and Measurement of Health for Adults in Health Insurance Study*. Vol. 1–VI. Rand Corporation R 1987/2, HEW., Santa Monica.

Stilwell, J.A. (1976) Benefits and Costs of the Schools' BCG Vaccination Programme. *British Medical Journal*, i, 1002.

Stourman, K. and Falk, I.S. (1936) "Health Indicex": A Study of Objective Indices of Health in Relation to Environment and Sanitation. *League of Nations Quarterly Bulletin of the Health Organisation*, **5**.

Strieenig, E.L. and Guttentag, M. (1975) *Handbook of Evaluation Research*, Sage, Beverley Hills.

Sullivan, D.F. (1966) *Conceptual Problems in Developing an Index of Health*, U.S. Department of Health Education and Welfare. Publication Number (HRA) 74–1017, Series, 2, Number 5, Dept. HEW, Washington D.C.

Sullivan, D.F. (1971) *A Single Index of Mortality and Morbidity*. HMSHA Health Reports, 347–55.

Swaroop, S. and Vemara, K. (1957) Proportional Mortality of 50 Years and Above. *Bulletin of the World Health Organisation*, **17**, 439–81.

Szabason, F. (1975) *L'Evolution de la Santé dans un Groupe Humain*. Dretoral Thesis of the University of Paris XI, Paris.

Szasz, T.S. (1961) *The Myth of Mental Illness*, Harper and Row, New York.

Tenhouten, W.D. (1969) Scale Gradient Analysis: a Statistical Method for Constructing and Evaluating Guttman Scales. *Sociometry*, **32**, 80–98.

Thienhaus-Grotjahn (1978) *Fruherkennung*, STE 22, Funkkolleg Umwelt und Gesundheit, Weinheim.

Thomas, L. (1975) *The Lives of a Cell*. Bantam Books, London.

Thurstone, L.L. (1927) Method of Paired Comparisons for Social Values. *Journal of Abnormal Social Psychology*, 21, 384–400.

Thurstone, L.L. (1931) The Indifference Function. *Journal of Social Psychology*, 2, 139–67.

Torgersen, W.S. (1958) *Theory and Methods of Scaling*. Wiley, New York.

Torrance, G.W. (1970) *A Generalised Cost-Effectiveness Model for the Evaluation of Health Programs*. Research Report Series 101, Faculty of Business, McMaster University, Hamilton.

Torrance, G.W. (1973) Health Index and Utility Models: Some Thorny Issues. *Health Services Research*, 8, 12–14.

Torrance, G.W. (1976a) Health Status Index Models: A Unified Mathematical View. *Management Science*, 22, 990–1001.

Torrance, G.W. (1976b) Towards a Utility Theory Foundation of Health Status Index Models. *Health Services Research*, 11, 349–69.

Torrance, G.W. (1976c) Health State Preferences: A Comparative Study of Three Measurement Techniques. *Socio-Economic Planning Sciences*, 10, 129–36.

Torrance, G.W., Sackett, D.L. and Thomas, W.H. (1973) Utility Maximisation Models for Program Evaluation: A Demonstration Application. In Berg (1973b), 156–65.

Torrance, G.W., Thomas, W.H. and Sackett, D.L. (1971a) *A Utility Measure of Effectiveness for Health Care Programs*. Paper to 39th National Meeting of the Operations Research Society of America, Dallas.

Torrance, G.W., Thamas, W.H. and Sackett, D.L. (1971b) A Utility Maximisation Model for Evaluation of Health Care Programs. *Health Services Research*, 7, 118–33.

Torrance, G.W. and Zipursky, A. (1977) *Economic Evaluation of Treatment with Anti-D*. Paper to Rh Prevention Conference, McMaster University, Hamilton, Ontario.

Truett, J. *et al.* (1967) Multivariate Analysis of the Risk of Coronary Heart Disease in Framingham, *Journal of Chronic Diseases*, 20.

Tuckett, D. (ed.), (1976) *An Introduction to Medical Sociology*. Tavistock, London.

Twaddle, A. (1974) The Concept of Health Status. *Social Science and Medicine*, 8, 29–38.

Tuoy, C.J. and Wolfson, A.D. (1977) The Political Economy of Professionalism: A Perspective, in Trebilock M.J. *Four Aspects of Professionalism*, Consumer Research Council Canada, Ottawa, 1977.

Ueberla, K. (1979) Was ist Normal in der Medizin? (unpublished).

Uhde, A. (1977) *On the Optimal Allocation of Resources to Health Care: Implications for Cost-Benefit Analysis*, Economic Papers, University of Bergen.

Verges, P. (1972) La Fabrication des Indicateurs Sociaux. *Economie et Humanisme*, July—August, 14—24.

Wann, T.T.H. (1976) Predicting Self-Assessed Health Status: A Multivariate Approach. *Health Services Research*, 11, 464—77.

Ware, J.E. (1976) Scales for Measuring General Health Perceptions. *Health Services Research*, 11, 396—415.

Weatherall, J.A.C. (1978) Congenital Malformations: Surveillance and Reporting. *Population Trends*, 11, 27—9.

Welford, C.F. and Wiatrowski, M. (1975) On the Measurement of Delinquency. *The Journal of Criminal Law and Criminology*, 66(2), 175—85.

White, K.L. (1982) Evaluation and Medicine. Paper given at the 1982 Conference at Wolfsberg on Economic and Medical Evaluation of Health Care Technologies, (chairmen, A.J. Culyer and B. Horisberger).

Whitmore, G.A. (1973) Health State Preferences and the Social Choice. In Berg (1973b), 135—45.

Whitmore, G.A. (1976) The Mortality Component of Health Status Indexes. *Health Services Research*, 11, 370—90.

Williams, Alan (1974) Measuring the Effectiveness of Health Care Systems. In M. Perlman (ed.), *The Economics of Health and Medical Care*, Macmillan, London.

Williams, Alan (1978) 'Need' — An Economic Exegesis. In Culyer and Wright (1978).

Williams, Alan (1979) One Economist's View of Social Medicine. *Epidemiology and Community Health*, 33, 3—7.

Williams, R.G.A. (1979) Theories and Measurement in Disability. *Journal of Epidemiology and Community Health*, 33, 32—47.

Williams, R.G.A., Johnston, M., Willis, L.A. and Bennett, A.E. (1976) Disability: A Model and Measurement Technique. *British Journal of Preventive and Social Medicine*, 30, 71—8.

Wilson, R. and White, B. (1977) Changes in Morbidity, Disability and Utilization Differentials Between the Poor and the Non-Poor: Data from Health Interview Survey: 1964 and 1973. *Medical Care*, 15, 636—46.

Wolfson, A.D. (1974) *A Health Index for Ontario*. Ministry of Treasury and Intergovernmental Affairs, Toronto.

Wood, P.H.N. and Badley, E.M. (1978) An Epidemiological Appraisal of Disablement. In Bennett, A.E. (ed.), *Recent Advances in Community Medicine*, Churchill Livingstone, London.

Woolsey, T.D. (1975) Using Statistics in Health Planning and Decision Making. In *Proceedings of the Public Health Conference on Records and Statistics*, DHEW Publication No. (HRA 74—1214), US Government Printing Office, Washington D.C., 21—6.

World Health Organisation (1957) *Measurement of Levels of Health: Report of a Study Group*. WHO Technical Report Series No. 137, World Health Organisation, Geneva.

World Health Organisation (1958) *The First Ten Years of the World Health Organisation*. World Health Organisation, Geneva.

World Health Organisation (1980) *International Classification of Impairments, Disabilities, and Handicaps*. World Health Organisation, Geneva.

Wright, K.G. (1974) Alternative Measures of Output of Social Programmes: the Elderly. In Culyer, A.J. (ed.), *Economic Policies and Social Goals*, Martin Robertson, London, 239–72.

Wright, K.G. (1978) Output Measurement in Practice. In Culyer and Wright 1978. 46–64.

Wyler, A.R., Masuda, M. and Holmes, T.D. (1967) Seriousness of Illness Rating Scale. *Journal of Psychosomatic Research*, 11, 363–74.

Wylie, C.M. and White, B.G. (1964) A Measure of Disability. *Archives of Environmental Health*, 8, 834–9.

Young, C.L., Chen, K.P. and Lan, C.P. (1974) A Survey of Physical Health in a General Population of North Taiwan. *Journal of the Formosan Medical Association*, 73, 8–15.

Zapf, W. *et al.* (1977) *Sozialer Wandel und Wohlfahrtsentwicklung in der Bundesrepublik, 1950–1975*. Sozialpolitische Forschergruppe Frankfurt/Mannheim.

Zola, I.K. (1966) Culture and Symptoms – An Analysis of Patients' Presenting Complaints. *American Sociological Review*, 31, 615–30.

Index